MEDITERRANEAN DIET

Mediterranean diet for beginners. complete guide. Everything you need to know to get started. How to Weight loss, following a healthy lifestyle, know their cooking history and learn delicious, quick and easy recipes.

BY
ROBERTO GIULIANI

Outline

- Introduction to the Mediterranean Diet

- History and Birth of the Mediterranean Diet

- What Exactly is the Mediterranean Diet?

- Guide to the Mediterranean Diet

  o Breakfast Inspirations for the Mediterranean Diets

  o Best food for lunch on the Mediterranean Diet

  o Food you Should Avoid on Mediterranean Diet

  o What You Should Keep in Mind Before Starting the Diet

  o How to Start and Stay on the Diet

- Benefits and Advantages of the Mediterranean Diet

- Exercises to Do with The Mediterranean Diet

  o How to Lose Weight on a Mediterranean Diet

  o Reasons You Are Not Losing Weight on the Mediterranean Diet

  o Lifestyle Lessons to Emulate with the Mediterranean Diet

- How to Set Your Goals for Weight Loss

  o Setting and Planning Weight Loss Goals

  o How to Lose Weight on the Mediterranean Diet

  o A Lifestyle for Good Health and Weight Management

  o Perfect Weight Loss Strategies

- Quick Recipes for the Mediterranean Diet

INTRODUCTION

The Mediterranean diet plan is a mix of the typical cooking styles of the countries encompassing the Mediterranean Sea, which extends from Spain, Italy, North Africa to the Middle East. An expanding number of specialists keep on showing with a lot of revelations that eating a diet wealthy in plant foods and high fats is good for the body. They said it helps fight against cardiovascular sickness, metabolic disorder, malignant growth, heftiness, type 2 diabetes, dementia, and Alzheimer's infection. These diseases have demonstrated to be the reason for a ton of deaths, anxiety, and disorders in human.

The regular American diet contains loads of sugar, fat, and salt. At the point when these three are all in a food plan, it makes for an unfortunate mixture. It can prompt weight increase, cognitive decline, and a large group of related wellbeing dangers. The Mediterranean diet, conversely, is high in lean protein, healthy fats, and vitamins and minerals. Best of all, the Mediterranean diet is more delicious than the American diet. It can only take some becoming acclimated to for certain people. Be that as it may, in case you're willing to attempt new things and train your body to incline toward familiar, supplement rich foods over-processed food that is stacked with saturated fat, you will before long be carrying on with a more joyful, more advantageous life.

The Mediterranean Diet isn't an eating plan, yet it's a way of life. The Mediterranean locale harbors probably the most loved food plans on the planet, yet additionally the absolute longest-living individuals. While the meal plans are significant, the diet moves the concentration from calorie tallying to a complete life change. This diet lessens the danger of heart illnesses. Also, it additionally sees to the prevention of Alzheimer's and Parkinson's infection through its demonstrated lower probability of psychological hindrance. In light of the propensities for the occupants of the Mediterranean Basin, this plan discovers its establishment in savoring and eating mostly natural products, vegetables, entire grains, and nuts. Different proposals of this diet incorporate standard physical exercises and activities and eating with family and companions, making this an extraordinary plan to appreciate with others.

The possibility of a Mediterranean diet has been around since the 1950s, when an American researcher, Ancel Keys, was doing exploration in Southern Europe. He saw that the individuals living around the Mediterranean, by and large, survived to a ripe old age. He also noticed that they had a much slower pace of heart and terminal illness than other regions of the world. This was in spite of a physically extreme, tasking, and challenging way of life and restricted funds. Keys inferred this wasn't incident or good karma, yet was identified with their diet. Ancel Keys saw that they ate more fish, grains, and vegetables - and he likewise recognized that the fat substance of the Mediterranean diet was altogether different. It was (and still is) much lower in 'awful,' saturated fats and higher in 'great,' poly-and mono-unsaturated fats. Fish shapes a unique piece of the diet - yet once in a while, battered or roasted. Although meat is eaten and eaten frequently, animal fat is once in a while utilized in cooking. Olive oil is generally employed. One of the most profoundly appraised diets by medical experts, The Mediterranean Diet, is frequently viewed as probably the best diet to live on as a lifestyle. It has been accepted as a significant aspect of an extended haul plan for wellbeing and wellness as opposed to a short-term plan to accomplish a specific weight loss objective.

What is it about this diet?

As it's been known previously, the Mediterranean diet is viewed as a conventional method for eating local to the individuals of the Mediterranean region. These regions comprise of countries, such as Italy, Spain, Greece, and Cyprus. The key benefit of the Mediterranean eating regimen is in the prevention of heart diseases. Over an extensive period, quite a while to decades, professionals have demonstrated that those that pursue the Mediterranean diet are fundamentally more averse to experience heart and other related diseases than those that don't. Heart ailment, Parkinson's illness, Alzheimer's disease, cancer and other associated diseases realized by terrible wellbeing and diet are among the most significant reasons for death in numerous urban populaces (USA, UK, Australia, Canada). A long-lasting adherent of the Mediterranean diet (and it is a deep-rooted diet) will be at a whole lot lower danger of these diseases than other people who are most certainly not.

History and Birth of the Mediterranean Diet

The Mediterranean eating regimen is an eating routine motivated by the dietary patterns of Greece and Italy during the 1960s. The vital parts of this eating routine incorporate relatively high utilization of olive oil, vegetables, foul grains, organic products, and vegetables, moderate to high usage of fish, reasonable use of dairy items (generally as cheddar and yogurt), fair wine utilization, and low utilization of non-fish meat items.

There is some proof that the Mediterranean eating routine brings down the danger of heart illness and early demise. Surveys in recent times have discovered that the evidence survives from low quality and is debatable. Olive oil might be the primary wellbeing advancing piece of the eating routine. There is a fundamental proof that ordinary utilization of olive oil may likewise lessen all-cause mortality and the danger of cancerous growths in the body cells, cardiovascular illness, neurodegeneration, and other dangerous diseases.

The Mediterranean eating regimen is approximately associated with the social practices, a lot of abilities, learning, customs, images, and conventions concerning crops, reaping, fish hunting, animal farming, protection of foods and plants, cooking, and especially the sharing and utilization of food, not as a specific arrangement of sustenance. Its supporters include Italy, Spain, Portugal, Morocco, Greece, Cyprus, and Croatia.

The Mediterranean eating regimen has its sources in a bit of land thought about one of a kind in its sort, the Mediterranean bowl, which students of history called "the support of society," in appraisal of the reality that inside its geological enclaves, the entire history and civilization of the old world took place. At its banks extended the valley of the Nile, the site of an antiquated and propelled progress, and the two incredible bowls of the Tigris and Euphrates, which were nature of the human growth of the Sumerians, Assyrians, Babylonians, and Persians. In the Mediterranean locale emerged the intensity of the Cretans. At that point rose the Phoenicians and the scholarly Greeks up to the developing strength of Rome. This enabled the region to turn into the "great land" between the East and the West. From that time, the Mediterranean turned into the gathering spot of individuals who, with their contacts, have now and then adjusted societies, traditions, dialects, religions, and perspectives about changing and changing the way of life with the advancement of history. The conflict between these two societies delivered their fractional coordination, so even the dietary patterns converged to a limited extent.

The starting points of the Mediterranean Diet are lost in time since they sink into the dietary patterns of the Middle Ages. However, in the old Roman custom - on the model of the Greek - distinguished in bread, wine and oil items an image of provincial culture and horticultural, enhanced by sheep cheese, vegetables (leeks, mallow, lettuce, chicory, mushrooms), little meat and a solid inclination for fish and fish. The affluent classes cherished the new fish (who ate for the most part seared in olive oil or barbecued) and fish, particularly oysters and prawns, eating it in its crude form or fried. Captives of Rome, be that as it may, were predetermined poor food comprising of bread and a large portion of a pound of olives and olive oil a month, with some salted fish,

9

once in a while a little meat. The Roman convention before long conflicted with the style of sustenance imported from the way of life of the Germanic people groups, chiefly travelers, living in close amicability with the timberland, got from the equivalent, with chasing, cultivating and assembling, the more significant part of the food assets. Raised pigs of fat, generally utilized in the kitchen, and developed vegetables in little gardens near the camps. The few grains produced were not used to make bread, but lager beer. The conflict of these two societies delivered their fractional reconciliation so even the dietary patterns converged to a limited extent. In any case, the Roman culture showed itself reluctant to change the style of Mediterranean Diet of encouraging with that of the barbarians. The critical components of the Mediterranean eating regimen, which is the group of three oil bread and wine, were sent out preferably in locales of mainland Europe by the ascetic requests, which moved in those districts to proselytize those people groups. Food, oil, and wine were in certainty the focal components of the Christian formality, yet they were later received likewise in the sustaining of the ordinary citizens of Europe. The new sustenance culture conceived from the association and the combination between dietary examples of two distinct civic establishments, the Christian Roman Empire and the Germanic, crossed with the progression of time with a third custom or that of the Arab world, which had built up its very own one of a kind food culture on the southern shores of the Mediterranean.

Just Muslims gave a lift to a restoration of farming that affected the sustenance model with the presentation of plant species known or utilized uniquely by the wealthier social classes, due to the high costs, for example, sugar stick, rice, citrus, eggplant, spinach and flavors, just as discovered use in the cooking of southern Europe, rose water, oranges, lemons, almonds, and pomegranates. Islamic culture, accordingly, takes an interest in the change and change of the social solidarity of the Mediterranean, which Rome had assembled, and gives a definitive commitment to the new culinary model that was framing. A noteworthy number of foods, gone by Muslims on Latin, drag their planning systems and plans.

Another occasion of extraordinary verifiable effect was, as it is outstanding, the revelation of America by Europeans. This revelation is likewise pondered in a buy the piece of the culinary convention of new staples, for example, potatoes, tomatoes, corn, peppers, and stew, just as various assortments of beans. The tomato, a natural decorative product just belatedly thought to be palatable, was the principal red vegetable that advanced our container of plants and later turned into an image of the Mediterranean cooking.

If the emphasis of vegetables is one of the unique characters of the Mediterranean convention, it is imperative to recollect the job of grains as the premise of basic cooking. Also, it is further necessary to see it as a weapon of everyday endurance, given their capacity to fill the stomach, diminishing cravings for food of poor classes. The kind of oats expended, just as the methods of change, accept various aspects relying upon the topographical undertones and customs that portray the populaces of the nations verging on the Mediterranean. Bread, polenta, couscous, soups, paella, and pasta are various approaches to devour oats.

This correct way portrayed permits distinguishing numerous similitude between the Mediterranean diet and current diet of our precursors to show the nearness of a genuine way that from the bolstering of the Egyptians to the disclosure of America prompted the presentation of new types of foods, giving us the Mediterranean diet as we probably are aware today.

The Mediterranean Diet is a healthful model, so all around valued that has a place with the social, correct, social, regional and natural and is firmly identified with the way of life of the Mediterranean people groups since their commencement. The Mediterranean Diet is a way of life and a lifestyle which means it is a social practice dependent on all the "savoir-faire", learning, conventions running from the scene to the table and covering the Mediterranean Basin, societies, collecting, angling, protection, handling, readiness, cooking and precisely the manner in which it is eaten.

The Mediterranean diet, referred to principally as a sustenance model, improves the quality and security of foods and their connection to the place that is known for starting point. It offers straightforward cooking, yet wealthy in the creative mind and tastes, exploiting all parts of a solid diet. It is a moral decision that jelly the conventions and traditions of the people groups of the Mediterranean Basin. Encouraging can significantly influence the wellbeing of people. This is because a decent nourishing status keeps up an adequate degree of welfare and counteractive action of metabolic diseases, for example, stoutness, diabetes, hypertension, and so on. The Mediterranean Diet which is an asset for manageable advancement, is significant for every one of the countries verging on the Mediterranean, to the monetary and culture impact the sustenance covers all through the area and the capacity to move a feeling of coherence and character for nearby individuals.

Even though the temperance of the Mediterranean diet has been upheld since the Renaissance, the reception of the menu outside the Mediterranean area has demonstrated troublesome yet not feasible. Endeavors at advancing dietary change have been investigated in the compositions of Europeans and Americans since 1614 when Giacomo Castelvetro, an outcast from Modena, Italy, distributed a book in England on Italian natural product, herbs, and vegetables. The chronicled reasons for obstruction by gatherings and people culture, class, sex, and human brain science are uncovered by posing the inquiry, "What does sustenance intend to individuals?" Particularly educational are bombed endeavors by benevolent late-nineteenth-century American reformers to hurry the digestion of recently showed up migrants by meddling with their dietary patterns. The foundation of the New England Kitchen, which gave economical Yankee cooking planned to Americanize poor outsiders, served uniquely to facilitate food dissemination organizes between California homesteads and urban focuses, enabling chiefly Mediterranean gatherings to eat their standard sustenance. Productive endeavors at change are additionally investigated, prompting the end that the fantastic kinds of the Mediterranean diet give the most obvious opportunity with regards to impacting individuals to forsake unfortunate foods for new vegetables, natural product, grains, and olive oil. The diet must be advanced, in any case, by restorative and nourishing specialists, yet additionally by individuals who can influence experts on cooking and specialists in promoting and showcasing.

13

A few different investigations have approved Keys' discoveries with respect to the great soundness of individuals in the Mediterranean nations. The World Health Organization (WHO) appeared in a 1990 investigation that four noteworthy Mediterranean nations (Spain, Greece, France, and Italy) have longer life expediencies and lower paces of heart illness and cancer than other European countries and America. The information is noteworthy because similar Mediterraneans now and again smoke and don't have regular exercise projects like numerous Americans, which implies that different factors might be mindful. Researchers have additionally precluded hereditary contrasts since Mediterraneans who move to different nations will, in general, lose their wellbeing points of interest. These discoveries recommend that diet and way of life are central locations. A recent report directed in France found that the pace of heart assaults and the pace of cardiovascular deaths were lower for the Mediterranean diet bunch than for a gathering of controls.

The Mediterranean diet increased more notice when Dr. Walter Willett, leader of the sustenance division at Harvard University, started to suggest it. Albeit low-fat diets were prescribed for a heart ailment, Mediterranean gatherings in his investigations had exceptionally high admissions of fat, chiefly from olive oil. Willett and others suggested that the danger of heart infection can be decreased by expanding one sort of dietary fat—monounsaturated fat. This is the kind of fat in olive oil. Willett's proposition conflicted with regular dietary proposals to decrease all fat in the diet. It has been demonstrated that unsaturated fats raise the degree of HDL cholesterol, which is once in a while called "great cholesterol" as a result of its defensive impact against heart ailment. Willett has additionally performed examinations corresponding to the admission of meat with heart sickness and cancer.

Willett and other specialists in Harvard, with the support of WHO worked together in 1994 and planned the Mediterranean Food Pyramid for the easy comprehension of the diet. This was meant to record the nutrition types and their suggested day by day servings in the Mediterranean diet. These nutritionists consider their nutritional categories an increasingly refreshing option in contrast to the dietary groups assigned by the U.S. Branch of Agriculture (USDA). The USDA suggests a lot of higher number of day-by-day servings of meat and dairy items, which Mediterranean diet masters ascribe to political factors instead of sound, wholesome examination.

This diet is a nourishing model dependent on the way of life of the individuals of the Mediterranean since their commencement - protecting their conventions and traditions and empowering things like occasional eating, moral decisions, and even reasonable improvement. As a diet, this model started expanding in fame with Western social orders after the 1950s. An American researcher, Ancel Keys, saw that poor populaces in the communities of southern Italy were by one way or another more beneficial than the majority of New York's wealthiest natives. To decide how this was conceivable, Keys set out on an investigation to determine the connection between these populaces to their diets - and the dietary benefit of the sustenance the Mediterranean individuals were expending.

15

This examination enlivened the principal "Sustenance Pyramid" discharged by the United States Department of Agriculture - a rule created to speak to a reasonable and adjusted method for eating. In any case, the handled and refined options in contrast to the regular foods devoured by Mediterranean populaces changed how the diet affected Western eaters.

The more present-day idea driving the Mediterranean diet perceives the destruction these foods can unleash on our bodies and energizes more advantageous, increasingly common choices - like those that would have been utilized by the antiquated Mediterranean human advancements. In the 1950s and '60s, when Americans were first setting out on a decades-in length, love-hate association with profoundly handled accommodation foods, Mediterranean towns (like those in Greece and southern Italy) were being read for their low paces of heart illness by the bespectacled and to some degree misjudged cardiologist Ancel Keys. Nourishing the study of disease transmission has advanced significantly since Ancel Keys' time, yet present-day networks that still hold fast to a conventional Mediterranean diet (in spots like Sardinia, Italy, and Ikaria, Greece) are being hailed as 21st century "blue zones," pockets far and wide where individuals live the longest.

Albeit new diets have moved toward becoming as flighty as design inclines, the Mediterranean diet – which highlights natural products, vegetables, entire grains, fish, olive oil, herbs, flavors, nuts, seeds, and some customarily delivered dairy – has stood the trial of time, proceeding to develop its awards among the food examine network. From heart infection and stroke anticipation, to sound loads and solid maturing, the Mediterranean diet is connected with an apparently perpetual rundown of potential advantages. Numerous parts of this healthy eating example are thought to help clarify its favorable circumstances, yet maybe the most critical trademark is its attention on entire foods as opposed to supplements.

By moving the accentuation from "fat" to olive oil and fish, or from "starches" to entire grains, products of the soil, disciples of a Mediterranean-style diet are allowed to search out healthy sustenances in the manner that nature planned. This methodology shuts a tricky dietary requirement, in which makers invigorate their items with some supplement, without really tending to the quality of the sustenance supply. Moreover, the Mediterranean diet is tied down by a sound base of social proof, as individuals have been experiencing these standards for a long time. The Mediterranean diet is perceived as a thing of an elusive social legacy by the United Nations Educational, Scientific, and Cultural Organization.

While the medical advantages of the Mediterranean diet were at first examined over 60 years back, the Mediterranean diet wasn't generally known outside the academic network until 1993, when Oldways banded together with the Harvard School of Public Health to make the main Mediterranean Diet Pyramid. So as to bring issues to light of the new kid on the culinary square, Oldways facilitated a progression of instructive meetings on the Mediterranean diet, and brought medicinal understudies, columnists and gourmet specialists on excursions directs to examine this eating design in situ, so they could spread the learning of this delightful and nutritious diet all through the United States.

Utilizing the richly shown Mediterranean Diet Pyramid as a guide, Oldways has helped the Mediterranean diet arrive at symbol status, showing customers and wellbeing experts the same that great wellbeing and great sustenance go connected at the hip. Scarcely anybody today could picture a solid diet without olive oil, verdant greens, hummus or if nothing else some trace of Mediterranean flair.

What Exactly is the Mediterranean Diet?

In agreement to what you've known so far about the eating regimen, A Mediterranean eating routine consolidates the general sound living propensities for individuals from nations flanking the Mediterranean Sea, including France, Greece, Italy, and Spain. The Mediterranean eating routine shifts by country and locale, so it has a scope of definitions. Be that as it may, as a rule, it's high in vegetables, organic products, vegetables, nuts, beans, oats, grains, fish, and unsaturated fats, for example, olive oil. It more often than excludes a low admission of meat and dairy sustenance. The Mediterranean eating regimen has been connected with high well-being, including a more beneficial heart. The Mediterranean eating lifestyle is generally a plant-based eating regimen, and professional dietitians and nutritionists have affirmed it with years of practical experience in the Mediterranean eating plan as a unique lifestyle that requires discipline, great exercise and sound way of life to make it compelling to the body framework. Likewise, this eating regimen has been known lately to be a worker diet in light of the idea of its birthplace, and a ton of elements joined to it. Individuals would eat whatever they had developing in their nurseries, alongside some dairy and olive oil.

For a helpful visual take a gander at the Mediterranean eating regimen of today, nutritionists have prescribed looking at the investigates done by Oldways, an association, alongside Harvard School of Public Health and the World Health Organization, that made the Mediterranean eating routine pyramid 25 years prior. On the activity stand the center sustenance: entire grains, natural products, vegetables, beans, herbs, flavors, nuts, and olive oil. The gatherings prescribe eating fish and fish two times every week and reasonable measures of dairy, eggs, and poultry. Red meat and desserts are expended just once in a while. How we consider "diet" today is something borne of confinement that causes you to get more fit. The Mediterranean eating regimen couldn't be further from that. Or maybe, it's a heart-solid eating regimen that incorporates the sustenance staples of individuals who live in the district around the Mediterranean Sea, for example, Greece, Croatia, and Italy. You'll see that in their suppers, they underscore a plant-based eating approach, stacked with vegetables and solid fats, including olive oil and omega-3 fatty acids from fish. It's an eating regimen known for being heart-sound. This eating routine is wealthy in products of the soil, entire grains, fish, nuts and vegetables, and olive oil. On this plan, you'll limit or keep away from red meat, sugary things, and dairy (however modest quantities like yogurt and cheese are permitted). Eating along these lines implies you likewise have no place for prepared admission. When you take a gander at a plate, it ought to overflow with shading; customary proteins like a chicken might be to a higher degree a side dish contrasted and the produce pressing the plate.

One thing you'll discover individuals love about the Mediterranean eating regimen is the stipend of reasonable measures of red wine. "Reasonable" here means 5 oz or less should be taken daily for the ladies which is about one glass, and close to 10 oz or thereabout, day-by-day for men should be taken which is about two glasses. To the exclusion of everything else, these suppers are eaten in the organization of loved ones; in number, social ties are a foundation of invigorating lives — and a stimulating eating routine. Here, food is commended.

When you consider Mediterranean food, your psyche may go-to pizza and pasta from Italy, or sheep hacks from Greece, however, these dishes don't fit into the sound dietary plans promoted as "Mediterranean." A genuine Mediterranean eating routine depends on the locale's conventional organic products, vegetables, beans, nuts, fish, olive oil, and dairy—with maybe a glass or two of red wine. That is how the occupants of Crete, Greece, and southern Italy ate around 1960, when their paces of ceaseless illness were among the most reduced on the planet and their future among the most noteworthy, in spite of having just restricted therapeutic administrations. Furthermore, the genuine Mediterranean eating regimen is about something other than eating new, healthy food. Day by day physical movement and imparting suppers to others are crucial components of the Mediterranean Diet Pyramid. Together, they can profoundly affect your mindset and emotional wellness and help you encourage profound gratefulness for the joys of eating well and tasty meal. Making changes to your eating regimen is once in a while simple, particularly in case you're attempting to move away from the comfort of handled and takeout food. In any case, the Mediterranean eating routine can be an economical just as a fantastic and excellent approach to eat. Changing from pepperoni and pasta to fish and avocados may require some exertion, yet you could before long be on the way to a more advantageous and longer life.

In reality, it's commonly acknowledged that the people in countries around the Mediterranean Sea live more and experience minimal effects of disease and cardiovascular illnesses. The not astounding mystery is a functioning way of life, weight control, and an eating routine low in red meat, sugar and soaked fat and high in produce, nuts and other invigorating food. The Mediterranean Diet may offer a large group of medical advantages, including weight reduction, heart and cerebrum wellbeing, disease counteractive action, and diabetes anticipation and control. By following the Mediterranean Diet, you could likewise keep that weight off while maintaining a strategic distance from interminable sickness. There isn't "a" Mediterranean eating regimen. Greeks eat uniquely in contrast to Italians, who eat uniquely in comparison to the French and Spanish. Be that as it may, they share a significant number of similar standards. Working with the Harvard School of Public Health, Oldways, a charitable food research organization in Boston, built up a customer well-disposed Mediterranean eating routine pyramid that offers rules on the best way to fill your plate – and perhaps wineglass – the Mediterranean style. The Mediterranean diet is certainly not a severe plan. Or maybe, it's a method for eating that stresses organic products, vegetables, entire grains, vegetables, and olive oil. Fish is the principle protein source rather than red meat, pork or poultry.

What's more, indeed, it incorporates red wine with some restraint. Matured dairy is devoured consistently, however in moderate sums. Eggs and poultry are at times expended; however, red meat and handled foods are not eaten routinely. The Mediterranean diet is related to lower cholesterol, diminished danger of heart illness and stroke, a lower risk of Parkinson's and Alzheimer's diseases, and a more drawn out life. Rising examination demonstrates it might likewise decrease danger of, and advantage those with, misery, uneasiness, type 2 diabetes, and a few diseases.

The establishment of this sound diet incorporates:

- an abundance of plant sustenance, including natural products, vegetables, entire grains, nuts, and vegetables, which are insignificantly handled, regularly crisp, and developed locally.

- olive oil as the chief wellspring of fat.

- cheese and yogurt, expended day by day in low to direct sums.

- fish and poultry, expended in low to direct sums a couple of times each week.

- red meat expended rarely and in limited quantities.

- fresh organic product for pastry, with desserts containing included sugars or nectar eaten just a couple of times every week.

- wine expended in low to direct sums, usually with suppers.

Individuals following the diet regularly cook these foods utilizing fortifying fats, for example, olive oil, and include a lot of delightful flavors. Suppers may incorporate little bits of fish, meat, or eggs. Water and shimmering water are necessary beverage decisions, just as reasonable measures of red wine. Individuals on a Mediterranean diet stay away from the accompanying sustenance:

- refined grains, for example, white bread, white pasta, and pizza batter containing white flour.

- refined oils, which incorporate canola oil and soybean oil.

- foods with included sugars, for example, cakes, soft drinks, and pastries.

- deli meats, sausages, and other handled meats.

- processed or bundled foods.

An ideal plate mirroring the Mediterranean diet is healthfully adjusted, differing, and loaded with shading, flavor, and surface. It's fresh, verdant greens; profound purple grapes; ruby-red salmon; energetic rainbow carrots; and nutty, crunchy farro. It's Greek yogurt bested with figs, dates, and a shower of nectar. Is your mouth watering? That is the point—the Mediterranean diet ought to never feel prohibitive. Instead, it's a scientific method for eating characterized by plant-based food, for example, vegetables, organic products, solid grains, vegetables, nuts, and seeds. In the United States, the Mediterranean diet's prevalence keeps on ascending close by a developing requirement for more beneficial eating examples and ways of life. The Centers for Disease Control (CDC) affirms coronary illness as the primary source of death in America for people, because of weight, terrible eating routine, absence of physical movement, diabetes, large amounts of awful LDL (low-thickness lipoprotein) cholesterol, and the sky is the limit from there. During the 1970s, U.S. physiologist Ancel Keys first connected a Mediterranean-style diet and better cardiovascular wellbeing through his "Seven Countries Study," however his hypothesis would not call on until a very long while sometime soon. During the 1990s, non-benefit Oldways Preservation Trust presented the Mediterranean Diet pyramid, offering Americans an alternate way to deal with smart dieting than the USDA food pyramid gave. Through vigorous research, expanded help from specialists, and proceeded with training to general society, the Mediterranean diet is viewed today as an incredible weapon against rising paces of coronary illness in the U.S.

Possibly the world's most beneficial method for eating, the Mediterranean diet depends on the customary sustenances that were devoured by populaces in Italy and Greece since forever. The food underscores products, fish, entire grains, and wellbeing fats - empowering a high admission of fiber, reduced utilization of meats and liquor, and vast amounts of cancer prevention agents. Adherents of this diet will likewise appreciate suppers with their friends and family - cooking as a family, eating as a family, and sharing a glass of red wine after supper as a family. Eating a lot of fresh, non-bland produce is vital to the Mediterranean diet. You'll need to go for in any event five servings every day, with each meal being around one cup of crude production. Solid fats are additionally empowered - originating from things like olive oil, nuts, fish, and avocado. Vegetables not just contain a considerable amount of these vital fats, yet include a robust increase in protein - and lean protein from non-meat sources is another foundation of this diet. To pursue the Mediterranean diet as suggested, plan to eat a serving of vegetables (a half-cup, cooked) in any event two times per week, and a little bunch of nuts each day. Protein from fish and eggs is additionally urged - a few times every week. Dairy protein, got from milk items like yogurt and new cheeses, ought to be expended day by day. Attempt to get one to three servings of dairy, one cup of milk or yogurt or one ounce of cheddar. Lean meats and poultry are welcome in the diet. However, these are to be appreciated with some restraint. Sugars are incorporated into this diet, also. Refined carbs, be that as it may, are disheartened - as these will cause issues with your glucose. Go for four little parts of entire grain carbs every day - whole wheat bread, pasta produced using quinoa, or grew or aged grains. This ought to consistently be overwhelmed by solid fats and protein, to guarantee legitimate assimilation and supplement ingestion.

You ought to likewise improve your dinners with fresh herbs and flavors, which are brimming with cell reinforcements and mitigating properties. Drink a lot of water, yet besides, espresso, tea, and even a glass of red wine every day. This diet is a nourishing model dependent on the way of life of the individuals of the Mediterranean since their commencement - safeguarding their conventions and traditions and empowering things like occasional eating, moral decisions, and even practical improvement. This region of the world is referred to by history specialists as "the support of society," since it is inside this locale that most of the old-fashioned development occurred.

As a diet, this model started expanding in prevalence with Western social orders after the 1950s. An American researcher, Ancel Keys, saw that poor populaces in the communities of southern Italy were some way or another more beneficial than the majority of New York's wealthiest residents. To decide how this was conceivable, Keys left on an investigation to determine the connection between these populaces to their diets - and the health benefit of the foods the Mediterranean individuals were eating. This investigation roused the primary "Food Pyramid" discharged by the United States Department of Agriculture - a rule created to speak to a reasonable and adjusted method for eating. Be that as it may, the prepared and refined options in contrast to the characteristic foods devoured by Mediterranean populaces changed how the diet affected Western eaters.

Guide to the Mediterranean Diet

Numerous eating regimens are portrayed by the foods you can't eat; however, this isn't the situation with the Mediterranean eating routine, an eating regimen that accentuates eating foods like entire grains, vegetables, vegetables, fish, and olive oil. Along these lines, numerous individuals find that the Mediterranean eating routine is progressively about including sound foods into their eating regimen, instead of limiting the "terrible" foods. The Mediterranean eating routine is something where you're permitted significantly more than Atkins or keto and a ton of these different eating regimens; that is the reason it works for many individuals. It has a decent assortment of foods, so individuals can pick what works for them.

How does the Diet Work? Since this is an eating design – not an organized eating routine – you're without anyone else to make sense of what number of calories you ought to eat to lose or keep up your weight, what you'll do to remain dynamic and how you'll shape your Mediterranean menu. The Mediterranean eating routine pyramid should help kick you off. The pyramid stresses eating natural products, veggies, entire grains, beans, nuts, vegetables, olive oil, and tasty herbs and flavors; fish and seafood at any rate two or three times each week; and poultry, eggs, cheddar and yogurt with some restraint, while sparing desserts and red meat for exceptional events. Finish it off with a sprinkle of red wine (if you need), make sure to remain physically dynamic, and you're set. The Mediterranean eating regimen isn't carefully characterized. Rather

27

than principles, there's a food pyramid intended to manage right dieting decisions.

At the base of the Mediterranean eating regimen pyramid are entire, natural plant foods: entire grains, organic products, vegetables, beans, nuts, and unsaturated fats like those found in olive oil and avocado. These whole foods make up the more significant part of what you eat on the eating regimen. There's no compelling reason to prepare every feast without any preparation. However, the eating regimen empowers lessening refined grains and other handled foods.

Notwithstanding organizing plant foods, the Mediterranean eating regimen recommends eating fish or seafood, in any event, two times per week, as these are the best wellsprings of heart-and cerebrum solid omega-3 fatty acids. On the off chance that you hate seafood, don't preclude the eating routine presently — chia seeds, flaxseeds, pecans, and soybeans are generally great wellsprings of omega-3s and fit into the Mediterranean eating regimen structure.

Dairy, lean poultry, and eggs make up another degree of the eating routine pyramid, alongside the free rule to eat these animal products in moderate proportions every day to week after week. Chicken sandwiches and cheese-filled omelets are excellent for consumption on the Mediterranean diet eating plan. However, it shouldn't be what you eat most of the time.

Red meat, desserts, and handled foods make up the tip of the pyramid and are the things you ought to eat least frequently. They're not off the table; however, they're at times foods that you don't eat each day on the Mediterranean eating routine. While positively not required, a glass a day for ladies and two every day for men is beautiful if your primary care physician says as much. Red wine has gotten a lift since it contains resveratrol, an exacerbate that appears to add a very long time to live – yet you'd need to drink hundreds or thousands of glasses to get enough resveratrol to perhaps have any effect.

Classes of the Mediterranean Diet:

It has been brought up that the Mediterranean Diet centers around REAL food that is found in the Mediterranean. It's something that has made it unique and rare. The following are our suggested sorts of foods type, instances of each, and substitutes on the off chance that you don't occur to live on Sicily or Santorini:

- Vegetables: Regular Mediterranean Diet staples are artichokes, arugula, Brussels sprouts, celery, and peas. However, indeed, any vegetable you appreciate is sufficiently adequate.

- Fruits: Figs, mandarins, tomatoes (no doubt it's a natural product), and pomegranate are typical to the territory, yet organic product like apples and oranges works as well. Don't eat 5,000 calories of sugar-filled leafy foods and fruits for what reason you're not getting the shape you desire.

- Whole Grains: Grain, buckwheat, oats, rice, and wheat, as crisp made wheat pasta, whole wheat bread, and pitas.

Entire grains are supported in pretty much every article on the Mediterranean Diet. When we state "entire," we mean insignificantly handled and are expended in altogether littler segments than you're likely used to.

- Legumes: Think beans and lentils: an incredible wellspring of protein and fiber that likewise happen to be flavorful. Hummus, a dish from the Mediterranean, is made out of the chickpeas (a vegetable).

- Dairy: Keep in mind that pyramid from a minute back? You'll see that dairy is higher up, which means to devour in littler amounts. Why? Since analysts were worried about saturated fat. With the Mediterranean Diet, dairy tends to originate from cheese like brie, feta, and parmesan, and Greek yogurt (however I expect there they call it yogurt).

- Fish: Fish are pressed brimming with Omega-3 fatty acids (excellent!), which will, in general, be insufficient in most American/Western weight control plans and has been connected to wellbeing ailments. Fish like cod are found in the Mediterranean; however, you could go with alternatives like fish or salmon as well.

- Poultry: Tidbit: Did you know there are approximately three chickens on Earth to each individual? About 20 billion fowl share the planet with us. I've been perched on that measurement for some time and was anxious to share. In any case! Feel free to eat your favored poultry, which could likewise incorporate turkey and duck.

- Healthy Oils: Olive oil. On the off chance that there is one explicit sustenance connected to the Mediterranean Diet, it's olive oil. Olive oil is touted for its monounsaturated fat, dissimilar to the immersed fat of state spread. Anyways, both are fine.

In What Frequency Should Each Category of Food be Consumed?

That is a decent question, and relying upon your amount of every classification, you might get more fit (the majority of this will be secured). Notwithstanding that, everyone does the Mediterranean Diet in an unexpected way:

- Some contend that dairy shouldn't be in the Mediterranean Diet by any stretch of the imagination since it contains saturated fat.

- Others would state red meat ought to be recorded above because Mediterranean dishes frequently incorporate sheep.

- Depending on which nation in the Mediterranean you pick, your "diet" will be altogether different.

Try not to get impeded in the subtleties of the authoritative opinion or the history, Instead, take a gander at the rundown of food above. Move your eating and go for enormous successes, by eating protein and authentic food as recorded above, and you'll be vastly improved off than you are at present.

Breakfast Inspirations for the Mediterranean Diets:

When you're following an eating regimen, it's anything but difficult to get into a morning meal trench. The Mediterranean eating routine accentuates eating bunches of organic products,

31

vegetables, entire grains, and solid fats like nuts, seeds, and fish. Joining these components to cause a tasty and filling breakfast to can give your day a genuine lift. Looks into have been made by nutritionists and specialists to distinguish the best things to have for breakfast when you're following the way of life of the Mediterranean eating regimen. These things will give a reasonable image of the adaptability of the eating regimen since breakfast is a significant part of one's nourishing wellbeing. The accompanying choices can be given a shot:

- Greek Yogurt Studded with Berries and Flax Seeds:

When you're in a rush and need a high-protein breakfast that won't keep you remaining at the stove, pick plain Greek yogurt with a sprinkling of berries. Greek yogurt is stressed such that makes it higher in protein than regular yogurt. Yogurt is likewise wealthy in probiotics, which are great microbes important for some real capacities. Guaranteed dieticians around the globe have agreed with the realities. Going for plain yogurt is prescribed while on the Mediterranean eating routine to maintain a strategic distance from included sugars. On the off chance that you need a touch of sweetness, you can consist of a light shower of nectar.

For an additional portion of goodness, include ground flaxseed. It's wealthy in omega-3 polyunsaturated fatty acids, which are critical for battling irritation in the body. It is continuously prescribed to add ground flaxseed supper instead of ordinary flax seeds since they are consumed better in the body. Greek yogurt is lower in sugar, wealthy in calcium and nutrient B-12. It likewise contains live societies, or probiotics, that can have various medical advantages, including controlling processing and boosting your safe framework. What's more, since it's wealthy in protein, it will keep you full for more.

A little parcel (like 5 ounces or less) of plain Greek yogurt (sans fat or low fat) with a bit of new organic product is a decent nibble choice, now and again. Attempt to discover natural Greek yogurt (plain, obviously) that has been appropriately stressed. A few producers add a thickening operator to yogurt, which doesn't give similar advantages.

- Overnight Oats are Tasty and Filling:

All your requirement for a supporting and heavenly breakfast on the Mediterranean eating routine is a bunch of oats and a couple of hours to save. Medium-term oats with a tablespoon of nutty spread and blueberries. It's easy to get ready, has progressively dissolvable fiber and cancer prevention agents, and is filling. To make this dish, absorb a part of oats either water, milk, or plant milk in the fridge medium-term.

- Indulge in an Early Morning Vegan Grilled Cheese:

In case you're searching for an unconventional breakfast treat, it is prescribed to attempt an entire grain veggie-lover flame broiled cheddar. It's easy to get ready and tastes debauched while as yet being plant-based. Join whole grain bread with a spread of Vegenaise outwardly, vegetarian cheddar (zesty or coconut-based), tomato, avocado, and a sprinkling of hemp seeds. Include a cut of vegetarian bacon in case you're in the mind-set.

33

- Whip Up Toast with Peanut Butter and Banana Slices for a Simple and Fun Breakfast:

Who might have believed that one of the most loved snacks of individuals holding fast to the eating routine is an incredible breakfast choice on the Mediterranean eating regimen? This straightforward and no-cook feast can be cobbled together in minutes and eaten in a hurry. With whole grain bread, you'll be eating more fiber and vitamins than in white bread, and that will enable you to fight off those early in the day munchies. Nutty spread offers those incredible, sound fats with its protein, and the banana will include some sweetness, more fiber, and potassium.

- A Whole Grain English Muffin with Greens and Bean Spread:

Another simple breakfast on the Mediterranean eating routine is choosing an English biscuit heaped high with entire food garnishes. It is prescribed to spread grain as a whole of English biscuit with bean spread before including a bunch of spinach and a poached egg. Any bean plunge will do here: hummus, dark bean plunge, white bean plunge. It will maneuver the sandwich together into a firm supper. With somewhat salty and tart flavor alongside its nourishing punch, it's an incredible sub for cheddar, which ought to be utilized just sparingly.

Poaching the egg will enable you to maintain a strategic distance from extra calories than other cooking techniques include, yet amp up the delightful protein. You can likewise swap in any green you like in case you're not an enthusiast of spinach; however, spinach is pressed with fiber, nutrient, and potassium.

- Almonds and Almond margarine are an incredible method to begin your day with protein:

Almonds are an essential tidbit and fixing in Mediterranean suppers from breakfast through to supper. They offer a filling and stimulating blend of protein, fiber, and solid fats to enable you to feel fulfilled. Fragmented or sliced almonds are a significant expansion to your oats, oat, granola, muesli, yogurt, ricotta or entire grain biscuits, while almond margarine is flawlessly sprinkled over entire grain hotcakes, waffles, and natural product. It is additionally great to utilize almond flour to make almond blueberry flapjacks that have more grit than renditions made with white flour.

- Egg Bites are the Ultimate:

Ranch fresh eggs are usually served at breakfast in the Mediterranean and are viewed as a sound method to begin your day. Two eggs have 12 grams of brilliant protein for supported vitality and are unendingly flexible. Consolidate eggs into your Mediterranean breakfast by garnish smoked salmon toast with a poached egg, scrambling them with feta cheddar and tomatoes, or munching on soup vide egg nibbles. Another tip from the Mediterranean: eat the yolks. Egg yolks contain fat which encourages you to stay fulfilled longer. Egg yolks are additionally wealthy in choline, a supplement that is required for mental wellbeing and helps transport supplements around your body. No egg white omelets here; the Mediterranean eating regimen centers around entire food.

- Avocados have healthy fats that will keep hunger under control:

Even though they're not local to the Mediterranean district, avocados do offer monounsaturated fat, which is a similar kind found in olive oil. These fats provide potential heart medical advantages and can help with satiety. Avocados are a decent wellspring of fiber at [approximately] three grams for each serving (33% of a medium avocado). Fiber additionally encourages you to remain full and helps keep your glucose levels increasingly steady, which is pivotal to balancing out weight, mind-set, and vitality levels. Even though dividing an avocado and eating it with a spoon is absolutely an alternative, you can likewise add avocado to smoothies, heated eggs, or even delicious oats.

- Coconut Date Balls are Good for Breakfast Treats:

These plant-based treats will fulfill a sweet tooth without depending on table sugar. They're additionally an extraordinary a bite to pack for a post-exercise center treat. To make this dish, join slashed dates, firm rice oat, a touch of maple syrup, and a pat of liquefied margarine. Fold the blend into balls and secured with destroyed, unsweetened coconut. Dates have a colossal measure of fiber (around 6.4 grams for a half cup) and the fiber will hinder the ingestion of starches into your circulation system. Dates have a massive amount of potassium and no sodium. Three date balls ought to likewise give you enough protein for your morning meal, and they store well for a few days refrigerated.

- A Whole Grain Bagel with Hummus and Cucumber is a Satisfying Breakfast Dish:

Consolidating entire grains with delicious plant protein makes for a filling and healthy supper to get you to lunch. It is additionally prescribed to include fixing of a little whole grain bagel with hummus and including some cucumber cuts for crunch and flavor. Hummus is a wellspring of sound fats, which will enable you to feel fulfilled longer. We add cucumbers here to help the veggie servings in the day. The vast majority don't eat enough, and adding them to breakfast is an incredible arrangement.

Best food for lunch on the Mediterranean Diet

Putting together up your very own lunch toward the beginning of the day spares heaps of money, but at the same time, it's direction more advantageous (advance away from the pizza). Lunch is a simple method to jump on a wellbeing kick, and keeping in mind that eating Mediterranean sustenance (every one of the tomatoes, lemons, feta, or falafels you can put on one plate), you won't miss those fatty subs one piece. You will be unable to fly set to Greece and back in your one-hour break, yet these delicious Mediterranean plans unquestionably satisfy the promotion.

- Lemony Orzo Salad

This rice-molded pasta reigns in the realm of convenient dinners. You've most likely had a lot moving at summer picnics, so why not prepare it for snacks all week? You can eliminate fixings as you see fit, in any case, as seems to be, it's pressed with new cucumber, red onion, chickpeas, basil, mint, spinach, and feta, so essentially flawlessness.

37

- Falafel Kale Salad with Tahini Dressing

Handcrafted falafel seems like an overwhelming throughout the day try. As a general rule, you can get these veggie-lover fellas ready in only 10 minutes. To begin, you'll be mixing chickpeas, onion, and garlic in a food processor, and afterward including cilantro, parsley, cumin, coriander, and red pepper drops. When you've wrapped cooking your falafel, your base serving of mixed greens is similarly as straightforward: kale (marinated in lemon juice), red onion, white beans, and jalapeño. The blogger calls attention to that kale is astounding for supper prep since it can hold awake for days (can't generally say the equivalent regarding spinach).

- Gluten-Free Mediterranean Pasta

On account of the innumerable options in contrast to wheat, sans gluten eaters don't need to abandon that pasta life. This formula uses dark colored rice noodles to go with its simmered eggplant and cherry tomatoes. Besides, if there are different sorts that you extravagant progressively, similar to a chickpea-or quinoa-based pasta, you can without much of a stretch swap those in.

- Classic Mediterranean Salad

A bowl of great Greek serving of mixed greens needn't bother with any organization—it's lovely enough all alone. Plan spinach, dark olives, cherry tomatoes, daintily cut up red onion, and the adored salty cheddar, feta. For a primary dressing to suit it, join olive oil, red wine vinegar, minced garlic, Italian flavoring, salt, and pepper.

- Mediterranean Lentil Salad

Lentils are a washroom thing that can indeed hold up to anything—stews, soups, and so on. This formula makes them star without anyone else with the assistance of red onion, radishes, celery, red chime pepper, parsley, and feta. The best part? You can have a significant bunch prepared in under 30 minutes, and it'll keep for a considerable length of time.

- Greek Turkey Meatball Gyro with Tzatziki

You needn't bother with a Greek giagiá in your life to ace the gyro. Rather than conventional sheep for the meat (which can get pricy), this formula subs in delectable turkey meatballs enveloped by a pita and bested with tzatziki. Everything shrouded in the dearest cucumber yogurt sauce is better—these are simply realities.

- Mediterranean Quinoa Bowl with Roasted Red Pepper Sauce

Not any more miserable, soaked lunch servings of mixed greens for you. A brilliant bowl of quinoa, cucumbers, feta cheddar, Kalamata olives, red onion, hummus, basil, and a spot of cooked red pepper sauce will have all your collaborators looking over in jealousy.

- Greek Shrimp Souvlaki and Farro Bowl

A bed of farro is an open canvas, and this present bowl has lemon and herb barbecued shrimp, ringer peppers, zucchini, tomatoes, and olives to jazz it up. The formula calls for entire grain farro; however, you can utilize quinoa or even dark-colored rice.

- Greek Lemon Chicken Soup

This soup plays consummately with avgolemono sauce (egg and lemon), which, if you've attempted it, is presumably on your top-foods list, as ever. The warm an incentive on it is incredible as well (so ideal for the workplace microwave).

- Lemon Parmesan Chicken with Zucchini Noodles

We generally love our zoodles loaded with garlic and lemon— the cheddar is only a reward fixing. All you should be prepared to feast prep is spread and dried oregano (which you likely as of now have), chicken, garlic, lemons, a juice of your decision, and a lot of Parmesan.

- Quinoa Stuffed Eggplant with Tahini Sauce

These thick eggplants are anything but difficult to ship and much more straightforward to prepare the morning of. Stuff yourself with everything that goes into these: quinoa, mushrooms, whole plum tomatoes, garlic, and handcrafted tahini. You'll wonder why you at any point made do with the serving of mixed greens bar.

- Bulgar Salad with Feta

Bulgar can without much of a stretch stand its ground as the fundamental dish in your lunchbox. This one is extra lemony and combines impeccably with all the best herbs: cilantro, mint, and parsley. Concerning the must-have besting, you have feta, which is first marinated in lemon get-up-and-go, garlic powder, and fresh oregano — hi, serving of mixed greens we had always wanted.

- Mediterranean Veggie Sandwich

At the point when all your preferred fixings become the headliner, you realize noon will be high. This sandwich, which is a plate of mixed greens between two cuts of whole wheat bread, has lettuce, grows, tomato, cucumber, red onion, disintegrated feta cheddar, and for its star: peppadew peppers (both sweet and fiery). Concerning spreads, attempt any hummus.

Food you Should Avoid on Mediterranean Diet:

Numerous diets are portrayed by the foods you can't eat, yet this isn't the situation with the Mediterranean diet, a diet that underscores eating food types like entire grains, vegetables, vegetables, fish, and olive oil. Along these lines, numerous individuals find that the Mediterranean diet is increasingly about including sound food substances into their diet, instead of limiting "terrible" food. The Mediterranean diet is something where you're permitted much more than Atkins or keto and a ton of these different diets. That is the reason it works for many individuals. It has a decent assortment of food, so individuals can pick what works for them.

In any case, there are a few types of food to attempt to avoid in case you're following the diet. Here are the seven types of food you

41

should try to stay away from while following the Mediterranean diet.

- Red Meat and Meat Intake Should Be Limited on This Diet:

The Mediterranean diet has a slight veggie lover point, utilizing creature protein more as a supplement to the food than a fundamental dish. Thus, on the off chance that you attempt the Mediterranean diet, you'll need to restrain all meat consumption — particularly red meat. As indicated by experts and professionals, red meat ought to be eaten only a couple of times each month on the Mediterranean diet.

- Processed Meats Shouldn't Be Your Top Pick:

You ought to likewise attempt to keep away from restored and handled meats, similar to bacon, salami, and frankfurter. If you do need a creature protein, try an omega-3 and protein-rich fish like salmon, mackerel, or fish. Fish is the primary [animal protein source] even over poultry.

- Try to maintain a strategic distance from included sugars however much as could be expected:

The Mediterranean diet does exclude a ton of added sugars; thus, included sugars ought to be constrained in case you're adhering to this diet. This implies avoiding treats, most prepared merchandise, and sugar and syrup-improved beverages like pop and fake juices. To get your sweet fix, attempt to eat the organic product or prepared merchandise made with leafy foods sugars like cinnamon and nectar.

- Hard Liquors Aren't a Major Part of This Diet:

If you drink liquor, it's ideal to stay with wine as opposed to hard alcohols. There isn't a ton of vodka and tequila on this diet. Permitting wine isn't an encouragement to drink a jug with each supper. On this diet, attempt to stay without any than one glass of wine a day.

What You Should Keep in Mind Before Starting the Diet:

For those considering receiving the Mediterranean diet, congrats! You're well on your approach to accomplishing various profitable medical advantages and expanded life span - and you'll be eating delectable, healthy foods with your companions and friends and family. This is an extraordinary way of life for anybody to focus on; however, there are a couple of things for you to remember as you start your adventure to living the Mediterranean way. These tips will enable you to remain on track and rapidly realize the stuff to keep up this reliable way of life.

-YOUR MAIN COURSE SHOULD NOT BE PASTA AND BREAD:

While this diet allows you to keep expending sugars, remember that Mediterranean individuals don't enjoy large dishes of bread and pasta how Westerners do. Instead, these dishes are beneficial pieces of the dinner. You won't get the numerous advantages from this diet if you keep eating enormous helpings of carbs, which will cause your glucose to spike and prompt expanded wellbeing concerns. A commonplace Mediterranean plate will highlight a piling part of vegetables and serving of mixed greens, a little bit of lean protein, a half-cup to one cup of pasta, and, at times, a bit of bread. Concentrate on genuine entire grains to profit by the protein, fiber, and magnesium in these organic sugars.

-IF YOU THINK IT IS EXPENSIVE, THEN YOU'RE WRONG:

Regularly, individuals are disheartened from receiving this diet on account of what they envision will bring an additional cost. Be that as it may, when you're eating more beans and vegetables rather than pricier meats, and building up your suppers with vegetables and entire grains, you'll wind up setting aside cash - rather than spending your food spending plan on bundled foods or cheap food.

With some strong feast planning, you'll even have the option to purchase as often as possible utilized things in mass - like olive oil, dark colored rice, and vegetables. Heaps of these dry fixings have a long timeframe of realistic usability, and additional plants can generally be solidified and defrosted for later utilization. There are vast amounts of approaches to make this diet work for any spending limit, so don't give things a chance to like an envisioned cost shield you from rolling out substantial improvements.

- DEAL WITH YOUR ADDICTIONS AND TEMPTATIONS TO GUARANTEE SUCCESS:

This diet isn't prohibitive; however, you do need to avoid unfortunate, handled foods if you need to accomplish the full medical advantages that the Mediterranean diet brings to the table. This is a comprehensive guideline that can enable you to keep up any way of life change, yet it is excellent to remember at whatever point you're setting out on a solid diet plan.

Before stocking your kitchen with solid, Mediterranean diet-affirmed foods, set aside some effort to experience your pantries and get out any handled garbage that doesn't add to your new way of life. These foods will serve to wreck you, so dispose of them by giving them to food banks or offering them to a sanctuary. At that point, head to the market with your shopping rundown and buy the things that will bolster your sound diet.

Additionally, if liquor is an enticement for you, you ought to abstain from including this part of the Mediterranean diet. While alcohol, specifically red wine, is supported with some restraint, if constraining yourself is an issue, it's smarter to keep it out of your diet totally as opposed to hazard visit overindulgence - or notwithstanding building up a problem.

-THIS IS A DIFFERENT WORLD REQUIRING A CHANGE IN LIFESTYLE:

While the food is an enormous piece of this diet, carrying on with your life in the Mediterranean style incorporates substantially more than merely that. Try not to plunk down for a supper before the TV - sit with your family and companions to appreciate a restful supper. This association and loosened up eating knowledge is presumably similarly significant for your wellbeing.

Not exclusively will you appreciate the organization of your friends and family, you'll eat all the more gradually and enjoy each nibble. This will enable you to figure out how to comprehend your body's sign - so you'll be bound to eat when you're eager and perceive that you should quit eating when you're full. You'll see

45

how to eat until you're fulfilled, rather than until when your plate is clean.

Mediterranean individuals additionally advantage from a lot of activity, so guarantee that you're getting enough physical movement every day. Park further away from your office or the store, take the stairs at whatever point conceivable and intend to go through at any rate twenty minutes daily doing the activity you appreciate.

How to Start and Stay on the Diet

A diet that is useful for sound weight reduction? Check. One that lessens the hazard for diabetes, elevated cholesterol, heart ailment, stroke, and a few fatalities? Check. A diet that reinforces bones improves mental wellbeing and averts dementia and sorrow? Check. As per logical research, that unthinkable list of things to get is satisfied by a diet regular to inhabitants of 21 sun-drenched nations that encompass the Mediterranean Sea. Even though it's known as the Mediterranean diet, it's not so much a diet since it doesn't reveal to you what to eat and not eat. It's a way of life that energizes devouring all nutrition types, however, gives more weight to those who have the most medical advantages.

- Focus on plants

That implies an accentuation on plants: organic products, vegetables, grains, nuts, and seeds. Eat a lot of veggies and utilize various types and hues to get the broadest scope of supplements, phytochemicals, and fiber — Cook, meal or trimming them with herbs and a touch of additional virgin olive oil.

Avoid coconut and palm oil even though they are plant-based; those oils are high in saturated fats that will raise terrible cholesterol. Add entire grains and natural product to each feast, yet utilize nuts and seeds as a trimming or little nibble because of their fatty and fat substance. On the Mediterranean diet, fish and other fish are devoured in any event two times every week. Cheese and yogurt appear day by day to week after week, in moderate segments; chicken and eggs are alright now and again; however, the utilization of different meats and desserts is restricted.

A diet where meat is as uncommon as desserts? For any individual who thinks a supper is worked around a segment of red beef, pork, or chicken, the idea of a plant-based diet can appear to be overpowering. It doesn't need to be a finished upgrade medium-term or be win or bust for you to begin to move your wellbeing. With regards to proper dieting, each nibble tallies.

-   Add happy development and mingle

Its central goal is to energize proper dieting employing the utilization of customary diets dependent on African, Asian, Latin American and, obviously, Mediterranean legacies.

As a visual method to empower change, Oldways made the Mediterranean diet pyramid in 1993, as a team with the Harvard School of Public Health and the World Health Organization.

Strangely, the ground level of the pyramid doesn't concentrate on food by any stretch of the imagination. Preferably, the best accentuation is set on exercise, carefully eating with loved ones, and associating over dinners. Masters empower in any event 20

47

minutes for each dinner. It is reasonable that that can be hard for many individuals to actualize, yet start little. Mood killer, the TV, set away from the mobile phone, center around meaningful discussions, bite gradually, and the delay between nibbles. That could be the beginning of your careful eating venture.

Concerning work out, it doesn't need to be in a rec center. The Mediterranean way of life is strolling with loved ones as opposed to considering exercise something that you need to do, walk or move or move in euphoric ways.

-   Move to entire grains

Perhaps the most straightforward advance to take when beginning the Mediterranean diet is to supplant refined grains with entire grains. Pick whole wheat bread and pasta, and replace white rice with dark-colored or wild rice. To ensure that what you purchase is in reality entire grain, Oldway's Whole Grain Council has built up a dark and gold "entire grains stamp" that makers can intentionally use, with each stamp posting the measure of entire grains in that item. The mark is on 12,000 items in more than 58 nations; customers can look through items by countries to discover what they need.

In case you're looking at two changed portions of bread, for instance, one may have 18 grams of entire grain per cut, and one may have 22, so in case you're new to whole grains, maybe you need to begin lower and stir your way up. Grains that have changed minimally throughout the hundreds of years, known as "old grains," are likewise a vital component of the Mediterranean diet. Quinoa, amaranth, millet, farro, spelled, Kamut (a wheat grain said to be found in an Egyptian tomb) and teff (an Ethiopian grain about the size of a poppy seed) are a few instances of old grains. Every one has an alternate taste and surface, so it is proposed that you ought to consider evaluating one per month at home or an eatery.

Mediterranean cooking has been a great pattern for some time now since it's entirely simple to test various Mediterranean grains and foods because these kinds of fixings have turned out to be so well known in standard eateries. At any rate six servings of grains, possibly more, are recommended every day, and in any event half of those ought to be entire grain. In case you're stressed over the impact of carbs on your waistline, it is best you take a gander at the more drawn out term benefits.

A ton of inquiries regarding these low-carb diets has been asked as of late. Because something may enable you to get in shape rapidly doesn't mean it was stable for your body to do it that way. You can get more fit by getting jungle fever as well; however, that doesn't mean you ought to do that.

- Rethink your protein

To augment the advantages of the Mediterranean diet, shifted wellsprings of protein are critical. You don't eat meat and poultry every day to get your protein prerequisites. Beans and lentils are incredible wellsprings of protein, also. They likewise give you fiber, vitamins, and a great deal of cancer prevention agents.

A simple method to begin is to prepare one feast every week dependent on beans, entire grains, and vegetables, utilizing herbs and flavors to include punch. When one night seven days is a breeze, add two, and assemble your non-meat dinners from that point. To do that effectively, it will be celebrated if you consider stocking your washroom with simple to-utilize fixings. A portion of her preferred protein sources are lentils, canned beans, and chickpeas. Lentils take just 25 minutes to cook on the stove, with no medium-term drenching required; canned beans and chickpeas only should be flushed before they can be prepared into soups and plates of mixed greens or used to make quesadillas or burgers.

When you eat meat, have modest quantities. For a basic course, that implies close to 3 ounces of chicken or lean beef. Even better: Use little bits of chicken or cuts of lean meat to enhance a veggie-based feast, for example, a pan-fried food. Two servings per seven days stretch of fatty fish, for example, salmon, herring, sardines, and tuna fish are an unquestionable requirement on the Mediterranean diet because of their high substance of solid omega-3 fatty acids, a vital aspect for bringing down your hazard for heart sickness. Indeed, there is a hazard some fish may contain mercury and different contaminants, yet the American Heart Association says that the advantages of eating fish exceed the dangers.

The affiliation recommends eating a wide assortment of fish to limit any antagonistic impacts. Shrimp, salmon, pollock, canned light fish and catfish will, in general, have the least degrees of mercury, the gathering says, while swordfish, shark, mackerel and tilefish have the most significant levels and ought to be maintained a strategic distance from, particularly by youngsters and pregnant ladies. Dairy items are additionally an incredible wellspring of protein. Having Greek yogurt for breakfast or a solid shape of cheddar as a bite is empowered on the Mediterranean diet, as long as it's with some restraint.

In the Mediterranean, cheddar is eaten in little amounts, for example, a sprinkle of ground Parmesan on a soup or vegetable dish, and not in a four-cheddar pizza kind of way.

- Don't skip breakfast

The Mediterranean plan supports breakfast; generally, your body thinks food is rare and eases back your digestion, adding to weight gain. Pick between whole-grain toast, bagels, pita or English biscuits, spread with delicate cheddar, hummus, avocado or any nut margarine. You can likewise substitute entire grain oat, for example, cereal or granola, with up to some drain, yogurt, and soy or nut milk. Add a little to a medium natural product or some berries, rather than organic product juice, as the fiber will help top you off. To make that totality last until lunch, the plan recommends including an egg, yogurt or bunch of nuts to the feast. In case you're not in a rush toward the beginning of the day, breakfast can be a lot bigger undertaking. A morning meal wrap, veggie omelet or frittata, or an entire grain hotcake with new berries and yogurt are on the whole significant decisions. You can likewise break new ground. Why not attempt extra soup or an upper plate of simmered veggies for breakfast?

Numerous individuals in the Mediterranean eat little platters of food for breakfast; a couple of olives, some cheddar, some nectar, and natural product, things like that.

- Rethink dessert

Day by day dessert inside a Mediterranean diet is additionally unique concerning the average American determination. Eating

51

organic produce that is in season is the pastry of decision in the Mediterranean district, as opposed to our common baked goods, treats, and cakes. On the off chance that you feel worn out on eating the crude crisp organic product, get imaginative. Poach pears in pomegranate juice with a touch of nectar, at that point diminish the sauce and serve over Greek yogurt. Flame broil pineapple or different foods are grown from the ground with nectar. Make a sorbet out of the organic product, including avocado (it's hugely a natural product). Stuff a fig or date with goat cheddar and sprinkle on a couple of nuts. Make a darker rice apple fresh or even an entire wheat organic product tart.

A few societies in the Mediterranean include a glass of red wine to their day by day supper. In case you're not a wine consumer, don't begin: Although research has customarily demonstrated a defensive advantage on heart infection and diabetes, ongoing examinations question that suspicion, and the jury's out on the endless benefits of liquor of any sort.

Be that as it may, if you appreciate vino, it's fine to treat yourself with a little glass of red wine at dinnertime as a component of the Mediterranean diet. It's likewise alright to include the incidental bread kitchen treat or other extravagance. No food is genuinely beyond reach. Individuals have this attitude of alright, I have to remove sugar, cut carbs out. I urge you to figure, 'what would I be able to add to my diet?' Where would you be able to include more products of the soil? Where would you be able to include more beans and lentils and entire grains? Where would you be able to add a portion of those solid fats? With the goal that's the mindset, I empower a progressively positive way to deal with doing solid practices.

Benefits and Advantages of the Mediterranean Diet

Considered by numerous nutrition specialists to be one of the most heart-sound methods for eating there is, the base of the Mediterranean diet is stacked with mitigating foods and based upon plant-based food sources and solid fats. Because of much inquire about, this specific diet can ensure against the advancement of heart illness, metabolic intricacies, gloom, cancer, type-2 diabetes, obesity, dementia, Alzheimer's, and Parkinson's. The best part is, even with these advantages, regardless it gives a chance to individuals to eat, drink and be happy.

Ever wonder why individuals from the Mediterranean area appear to be so upbeat and brimming with life? It's enticing to trait their great wellbeing and positive states of mind to one single factor alone — like their diet, for instance — however in all actuality it's a mix of their way of life factors and their natural foods that have advanced their life span and low paces of infection for quite a long time.

It's been demonstrated that together with customary physical action and not enjoying smoking, more than 80 percent of coronary heart sickness, 70 percent of stroke, and 90 percent of type 2 diabetes can stay away from by reliable food decisions that are steady with the conventional Mediterranean diet. These examinations have turned out to demonstrate to be consistent with the life span of individuals occupying the Mediterranean district.

Thinking about what precisely it resembles to pursue this time tested eating plan, and what the Mediterranean diet advantages are? The most significant advantage of the Mediterranean diet (furthermore, you know, wine) is that it's well-considered making its hummed about benefits genuine. The Mediterranean diet has been around for an extremely, long time and is one of the eating plans that has been examined the most. A great deal of hypothesizes and research papers have been distributed from the investigation of this diet as far back as perusing and composing have been in presence. It indeed demonstrated the extended haul benefits, and that made it genuinely start flooding in prevalence. After some time, ponders have been done on the individuals who pursue the diet carefully and it has been found that the individuals who ate a Mediterranean diet had fundamentally less cardiovascular issues than the individuals who didn't. In any case, you can't generally say there's one uniform Mediterranean way of life or eating design since its adherents don't live in a similar spot. That muddles the push to survey the potential medical advantages of the diet. Did you live in Italy? Did you live in Greece? Did you live in Spain? Did you live in North Africa? So at that point, when you do research thinks about, the diet may be somewhat unique in each.

Likewise, eating and drinking with some restraint might be more diligently for those living on this side of the Atlantic to receive, mainly because the Mediterranean diet doesn't set calorie admission rules. It's a worry that somebody from the United States will attempt to include a quarter cup of olive oil to their diet, yet they're not going to remove a portion of the desserts and afterward they will get an excessive number of calories. Without restricting your intake to any boundaries, you can appreciate an improved personal satisfaction and expanded sentiments of prosperity on account of this sound, nutritious food. You'll see a vast amount of incredible advantages once you start eating Mediterranean-style - particularly influencing your heart wellbeing, mental wellbeing, and life span. These are only a portion of the manners in which your body and mind will profit by eating Mediterranean-diet endorsed foods. Here are the advantages of the Mediterranean Diet:

- Low in Processed Foods and Sugar:

The diet fundamentally comprises of foods and fixings that are near nature, including olive oil, vegetables like peas and beans, organic products, vegetables, grungy grain items, and little parts of creature items (that are always "natural" and privately delivered). Rather than the run of the American mill diet, it's deficient in sugar and free of all GMOs or counterfeit fixings like high fructose corn syrup, additives and flavor enhancers. For something sweet, individuals in the Mediterranean appreciate the organic product or little amounts of custom-made treats made with simple sugars like nectar.

Past plant foods, another real staple of the diet is privately gotten fish and a moderate utilization of dairy animals, goat or sheep cheeses and yogurts that are incorporated as an approach to get healthy fats and cholesterol. Fish like sardines and anchovies are a focal piece of the diet, which as a rule is generally lower in meat items than many Western foods today.

While a great many people in the Mediterranean aren't veggie lovers, the diet advances just a little utilization on meats and more massive dinners — instead of going for the lighter and more beneficial fish choices no matter how you look at it. This can be advantageous for those hoping to shed pounds and improve things, for example, their cholesterol, heart wellbeing, and omega-3 fatty corrosive admission.

- Helps You Lose Weight in a Healthy Way:

In case you're hoping to get thinner without being ravenous and keep up that weight in a reasonable manner that can endure forever, this may be the plan for you. The diet is both practical and advantageous and has been attempted by numerous individuals all around the globe with extraordinary achievement identified with weight reduction, and the sky is the limit from there, as it tries to help oversee weight and decrease fat admission regularly and effectively because of eating numerous supplement thick foods.

There's space for translation in the Mediterranean diet, regardless of whether you like to eat lower carb, lower protein, or someplace in the middle. The food centers around the utilization of sound fats while keeping sugars moderately low and improving an individual's admission of top-notch protein foods. If you allude protein over vegetables and grains, you have the alternative to shed pounds in a stable, no-hardship sort of-path with a high measure of fish and quality dairy items (that at the same time give different advantages like omega-3s and regularly probiotics). Fish, dairy items and grass-sustained/unfenced meats contain solid fatty acids that the body needs, attempting to enable you to feel full, oversee weight gain, control glucose, and improve your state of mind and vitality levels. Be that as it may, in case you're to a greater extent a plant-based eater, vegetables and entire grains (particularly if they're doused and grew) likewise make great, filling decisions.

57

Likely because of its emphasis on entire, new foods, the Mediterranean diet may enable you to get in shape in a sheltered and economical way, yet in case you're searching for quick outcomes, you might be in an ideal situation with an alternate diet plan. As referenced, in its 2019 rankings, U.S. News and World Report evaluated the Mediterranean diet as No. 1 in its Best Diets Overall class, yet the diet tied with a few different plans for the seventeenth situation among the site's Best Weight Loss Diets.

Over five years, eating a calorie-unlimited Mediterranean diet high in unsaturated vegetable fat prompted marginally more weight reduction and added less to members' midriff boundaries than a low-fat diet. Primarily, individuals who added extra-virgin olive oil to their foods lost the most weight — 0.88 kilograms (kg), or 1.9 pounds (lbs) by and large. The individuals who included nuts lost 0.4 kg normal (0.88 lbs), and those in the control bunch who ate a low-fat diet lost 0.6 kg (1.3 lbs).

When you include calorie confinement, the Mediterranean diet may demonstrate increasingly emotional outcomes, however not prevailing over another prevalent diet approach. In a two-year randomized, clinical preliminary, 322 modestly stout moderately aged members in Israel, who were for the most part men, tailed one of three diets: a calorie-confined low-fat diet, a calorie-limited Mediterranean diet, and a calorie-unlimited low-carb diet. Among the Mediterranean diet adherents, ladies ate a limit of 1,500 calories for every day, while men's carbohydrate content was confined to 1,800 calories for every day, to have close to 35 percent of their calories from fat. The calorie confinements were the equivalent for those on the low-fat diet. The mean weight reduction was 4.4 kg (9.7 lbs) for the Mediterranean-diet gathering,

2.9 kg (6.4 lbs) for the low-fat meeting, and 4.7 kg (10.3 lbs) for the low-starch conference.

- Improves Heart Health:

Research demonstrates that more prominent adherence to the conventional Mediterranean diet, including a lot of monounsaturated fats and omega-3 foods, is related to a noteworthy decrease on the whole reason mortality, particularly heart infection. A striking defensive impact of a Mediterranean diet wealthy in alpha-linolenic corrosive (ALA) from olive oil has been appeared in numerous examinations, with some finding that a Mediterranean-style food can diminish the danger of cardiovascular passing by 30 percent and unexpected heart demise by 45 percent.

Research from the Warwick Medical School additionally demonstrates that when hypertension is thought about between individuals eating more sunflower oil and those devouring all the more extra-virgin olive oil, the olive oil diminishes pulse by altogether higher sums. Olive oil is additionally helpful for bringing down hypertension since it makes nitric oxide increasingly bioavailable, which improves it ready to keep corridors expanded and clear. Another defensive component is that it helps battle the malady advancing impacts of oxidation and improves endothelial capacity. Remember that low cholesterol levels are more terrible than high now and then, yet individuals in the Mediterranean don't for the most part battle to keep up sound cholesterol levels either since they acquire a lot of solid fats. Various investigations propose the Mediterranean diet is useful for your ticker, noticed a meta-examination distributed in November 2015 in the diary Critical Reviews in Food Science and Nutrition.

For around five years, creators pursued 7,000 ladies and men in Spain who had type 2 diabetes or a high chance for cardiovascular ailment. The individuals who ate a calorie-unhindered Mediterranean diet with extra-virgin olive oil or nuts had a 30 percent lower danger of heart occasions. Analysts didn't exhort members on exercise.

The examination creators reanalyzed the information at a later point to address a broadly scrutinized defect in the randomization convention, and detailed comparative outcomes in June 2018 in the New England Journal of Medicine. That is most likely the most significant logical proof to state that a Mediterranean diet is therapeutic, as far as diminishing the danger of cardiovascular infection.

- Helps Fight Cancer:

A plant-based diet, one that incorporates loads of foods grown from the ground, is the foundation of the Mediterranean diet, which can help battle cancer in about each manner — giving cancer prevention agents, shielding DNA from harm, halting cell change, bringing down aggravation and postponing tumor development. Numerous investigations point to the way that olive oil may likewise be asymptomatic cancer treatment and lessening the danger of colon and gut cancers. It may protectively affect the improvement of cancer cells because of brought down aggravation and diminished oxidative worry, in addition to its propensity to advance adjusted glucose and a more beneficial weight.

- Prevents or Treats Diabetes:

Proof recommends that the Mediterranean diet fills in as a mitigating dietary example, which could help battle diseases identified with ceaseless aggravation, including metabolic disorder and type 2 diabetes. One explanation the Mediterranean diet may be so valuable for anticipating diabetes is because it controls overabundance insulin, a hormone that regulates glucose levels, makes us put on weight and keeps the weight stuffed on notwithstanding us dieting.

By directing glucose levels with an equalization of entire foods — containing solid fatty acids, quality wellsprings of protein and a few starches that are low in sugar — the body consumes fat all the more productively and has more vitality as well. A low-sugar diet with a lot of crisp produce and fats is a piece of a specific diabetic diet plan.

As per the American Heart Association, the Mediterranean diet is higher in fat than the standard American diet, yet lower in saturated fat. It's typically approximately a proportion of 40 percent complex sugars, 30 percent to 40 percent sound fats and 20 percent to 30 percent quality protein foods. Since this equalization is to some degree perfect as far as monitoring weight addition and appetite, it's a decent route for the body to stay in hormonal homeostasis, so somebody's insulin levels are standardized. As a result, it additionally implies somebody's state of mind is bound to remain positive and loose, vitality step up, and physical action simpler.

The Mediterranean diet is low in sugar since the primary sugar presents more often than not originates from the natural product, wine, and the incidental privately made sweet. With regards to drinks, numerous individuals drink a lot of crisp water, some espresso and red wine, as well. Be that as it may, pop and improved beverages aren't so well known as they are in the U.S.

While some Mediterranean diets do incorporate a decent arrangement of starches — like pasta or bread, for instance — being dynamic and generally expending shallow degrees of sugar implies that insulin opposition stays uncommon in these nations. The Mediterranean style of eating avoids tops and valleys in glucose levels, which destroys vitality and negatively affects your mindset. These different components add to this present diet's diabetes counteractive action capacities.

The vast majority in the Mediterranean have a fair breakfast inside one to two hours of awakening, which starts their day directly by adjusting glucose when it's at its most reduced. They at that point normally eat three suppers per day that are filling, with a lot of fiber and solid fats. Numerous individuals have their greatest supper noontime instead of around evening time, which offers them the chance to utilize that food for vitality while they're as yet dynamic.

You can perceive how this varies from the standard American diet, which frequently brings about numerous individuals skipping breakfast, eating for the day on vitality destroying foods high in carbs and sugar, and eating a ton at evening time while they're stationary.

- **Protects Cognitive Health and Can Improve Your Mood:**

Eating the Mediterranean way may be a specific Parkinson's infection treatment, an incredible method to preserve your memory, and a positive development for frequently treating Alzheimer's sickness and dementia. The intellectual issue can happen when the mind isn't getting an adequate measure of dopamine, a significant substance important for appropriate body developments, disposition guideline, and thought handling.

Solid fats like olive oil and nuts, in addition to a lot of mitigating veggies and organic products, are known to battle age-related subjective decrease. These enable counter the unsafe impacts of introduction to poisonous quality, to free radicals, aggravation causing less than stellar eating routines or food hypersensitivities, which would all be able to add to disabled mind work. This is one motivation behind why adherence to the Mediterranean diet is connected with lower paces of Alzheimer's. Probiotic foods like yogurt and kefir likewise help manufacture a solid gut, which we currently know is attached to intellectual capacity, memory, and temperament issue.

As a heart-sound diet, the Mediterranean eating example may likewise diminish a decrease in your memory and thinking abilities with age. The mind is an eager organ. To supply those supplements and oxygen [that it needs], you must have an abundant blood supply. In this way, individuals who are having any issues with their vascular wellbeing — their veins — are genuinely at expanded hazard for creating problems with their mind, and afterward that as often as possible will introduce itself as intellectual decrease.

63

A July 2016 survey distributed in the diary Frontiers in Nutrition took a gander at the impact of the Mediterranean diet on psychological capacity and finished up "there is empowering proof that higher adherence to a Mediterranean diet is related with improving cognizance, easing back intellectual decrease, or diminishing the transformation to Alzheimer's sickness. Also, a little report financed by the National Institute on Aging and distributed in May 2018 in the diary Neurology saw cerebrum checks for 70 individuals who had no indications of dementia at the beginning and scored them for how intently their eating examples slashed to the Mediterranean standard. The individuals who scored low would, in general, have increasingly beta-amyloid stores (protein plaques in the cerebrum related with Alzheimer's infection) and lower vitality use in the mind toward the finish of the investigation. At any rate two years after the fact, these people additionally demonstrated a more prominent increment of stores and decrease of vitality use — possibly flagging an expanded hazard for Alzheimer's — than the individuals who all the more intently pursued the Mediterranean diet.

All that stated, more research is required before prescribing this eating way to deal with lower Alzheimer's hazard. The creators needed extra explore in a more significant member gathering and for a more drawn out investigation period.

For the time being, the Mediterranean diet can be recognized as one method for eating that can help fight off subjective decrease. It's not suggested over other well-examined foods, for example, the MIND diet (MIND represents Mediterranean–DASH Diet Intervention for Neurodegenerative Delay), which is a crossbreed of the Mediterranean model and the circulatory strain bringing down DASH diet.

- Might Help You Live Longer:

A diet high in crisp plant foods and solid fats is by all accounts the triumphant mix for life span. Monounsaturated fat, the type found in olive oil and a few nuts, is the fundamental fat source in the Mediterranean diet. Again and again, thinks about demonstrate that monounsaturated fat is related with lower levels of heart illness, cancer, wretchedness, subjective decay and Alzheimer's sickness, provocative diseases and that's only the tip of the iceberg. These are presently the primary sources of death in created countries — particularly heart infection.

In the celebrated Lyon Diet Heart Study, individuals who had heart assaults somewhere in the range of 1988 and 1992 were either guided to adhere to the standard post-heart assault diet exhortation, which lessens saturated fat extraordinarily, or advised to pursue a Mediterranean style. After around four years, follow-up results demonstrated that individuals on the Mediterranean diet experienced 70 percent less heart infection — which is around multiple times the decrease in hazard accomplished by most cholesterol-bringing down remedy statin drugs! The individuals on the Mediterranean diet likewise incredibly encountered a 45 percent lower danger of all-cause demise than the gathering on the standard low-fat diet.

These outcomes were genuine despite the fact that there wasn't quite a bit of an adjustment in cholesterol levels, which discloses to you that heart malady is about something other than cholesterol.

65

The aftereffects of the Lyon Study were so great and noteworthy that the investigation must be halted ahead of schedule for moral reasons, so all members could pursue the higher-fat Mediterranean-style diet and harvest its life span advancing settlements.

- Helps Your De-stress and Relax:

Another affecting component is that this diet urges individuals to invest energy in nature, get great rest and meet up to bond over a home-prepared substantial dinner, which are extraordinary approaches to assuage pressure and, accordingly, help avert irritation. For the most part, individuals in these areas make a point to invest a great deal of energy outside in nature; eating food encompassed by family and companions (as opposed to alone or in a hurry); and set aside time to chuckle, move, nursery and practice side interests.

We, as a whole, realize that constant pressure can slaughter your quality your life alongside your weight and wellbeing. The individuals who practice the diet have the advantage of lazy feasting at a moderate pace, eating nearby delectable foods consistently and participating in regular physical movement as well — other significant variables that help keep up a cheerful state of mind.

Also, the historical backdrop of the Mediterranean diet incorporates an affection for and interest with wine — particularly red wine, which is viewed as valuable and defensive with some restraint. For example, red wine may help battle heftiness, among different advantages. This savvy decision of a healthy lifestyle prompts longer lives free of ceaseless intricacies and diseases identified with pressure, for example, those brought about by awkward hormonal nature, fatigue, aggravation, and weight gain. While following a Mediterranean diet, you ought to likewise hope to embrace different parts of the Mediterranean way of life - like making supper time an increasingly social encounter and investing more energy practicing and getting outside. These exercises hugely affect your wellbeing, more than you may suspect. You'll be eating nutritious sound foods, and profiting by an increasingly positive way of life. This way of life can give you better apparatuses to deal with life's numerous burdens, leaving you feeling frequently playful, loose, and revived. The constant pressure can be extraordinarily harming to your general wellbeing and prosperity, yet the Mediterranean diet can enable you to ward it off. You'll rest better, appreciate more vitality, and even form increasingly generous associations with your friends and family. Individuals who experience the ill effects of emotional wellbeing concerns like uneasiness, sadness, and even ADHD can appreciate a portion of the mind boosting advantages of the Mediterranean diet. These scatters can happen when your cerebrum isn't getting enough dopamine, which is the concoction in charge of idea handling, body developments, and disposition guideline.

Be that as it may, the solid fats and probiotic foods included and supported through this eating plan help your body produce this synthetic - keeping your disposition raised and your mind cheerful. They'll additionally add to gut wellbeing, which is a noteworthy trigger for temperament issue.

While specialists prescribe that individuals proceed with ordinary treatment programs, exchanging up your diet to receive a

Mediterranean way of life can be a fabulous enhancement to conventional treatments. With time, you may find that you never again require pharmacological obstruction.

- Can Help Fight Depression:

A recent report distributed in the diary Molecular Psychiatry discovered proof that reliable dietary decisions, those following eating the Mediterranean diet, can help decrease the hazard for gloom. Researchers associated with the examination explored the emotional being wellbeing impacts of adherence to a scope of foods — including the Mediterranean diet, the Healthy Eating Index (HEI), the Dietary Approaches to Stop Hypertension diet (DASH diet), and the Dietary Inflammatory Index. They found that the danger of melancholy was decreased the most when individuals pursued a conventional Mediterranean diet and in general, ate an assortment of mitigating foods.

What is it about calming foods that helps support your temperament and emotional wellness? Aggravation is much of the time named as the underlying driver of numerous states of mind and mental conditions, including schizophrenia, over the top urgent issue, sadness, uneasiness, fatigue, and social withdrawal. A similar way of life propensities that will, in general, actuate irritation, for example, a terrible eating routine, constant pressure and lack of sleep — additionally will in general produce cerebrum expresses that add to dysfunctional behavior. A thick supplement diet appears to help straightforwardly ensure portions of the cerebrum, while other dietary/way of life changes like getting excellent rest, having a careful approach to deal with dinners, planning suppers early, and constraining pressure can likewise prompt a quieter outlook.

The Mediterranean method for eating is connected to bring down the rate of discouragement, as per an examination of 41 observational investigations distributed in September 2018 in the diary Molecular Psychiatry. Survey of pooled information from four longitudinal studies uncovered that the diet was related with a 33 percent decreased danger of melancholy, contrasted and following a "star provocative diet" (more extravagant in handled meats, sugar, and trans fats) that is increasingly ordinary of a standard American diet. While the examination didn't uncover why a Mediterranean diet brought down sorrow chance, the investigation creators composed that their outcomes might be a starting point to create and read diet-based mediations for melancholy.

- Eating a Mediterranean Diet May Reduce Women's Risk for Stroke:

It is outstanding from past investigations that eating in a Mediterranean manner can help bring down the danger of cardiovascular illness in specific individuals. The diet may likewise help diminish stroke chance in ladies; however, researchers didn't watch similar outcomes in men.

Researchers took a gander at an overwhelmingly white gathering of 23,232 people ages 40 to 77 who lived in the United Kingdom. The more firmly a lady pursued a Mediterranean diet, the lower her danger of having a stroke. Be that as it may, researchers didn't see measurably remarkable outcomes in men. Most strikingly, in ladies who were at danger of having a stroke, following the diet diminished their odds of this wellbeing occasion by 20 percent.

Study creators don't have the foggiest idea about the purpose behind the distinction; however, they speculate that various types of strokes in people may assume a job. A decent subsequent stage toward understanding the explanations for the differences would be a clinical preliminary.

- Mediterranean Diet to Better Memory in Diabetics

Devouring foods and supplements regular for the Mediterranean dietary example has been reliably connected with better intellectual capacity among grown-ups and more seasoned adults. As expending a Mediterranean diet has been related to anticipation and control of Type 2 diabetes, this dietary example may have double benefits for both Type 2 diabetes and discernment. In the different examinations, the exploration groups pursued 465 grown-ups with Type 2 diabetes and 711 adults without the infection. The members were taken a crack at the Boston Puerto Rican Health Study from 2004 to 2007.

Utilizing food polls at a pattern and the two-year point, the researchers assessed adherence to the accompanying eating plans: MedDiet, Dietary Approaches to Stop Hypertension, Healthy Eating Index, and Alternative Healthy Eating Index. What's more, they observed blood glucose and surveyed intellectual capacity utilizing seven neuropsychological tests.

The outcomes demonstrated a connection between stricter adherence to the MedDiet and more advantageous comprehension for Type 2 diabetics at two years in contrast with the gauge. In any case, this advantage was just noted in members with stable glucose levels. At the point when the people had poor or declining blood glucose control, the connection vanished.

It's essential to take note of that the advantages of the MedDiet over other solid diets were noted uniquely among patients with Type 2 diabetes. Among those without Type 2 diabetes, every sound diet similarly improved memory work. Two variables may underlie the intellectual advantages of the MedDiet in patients with Type 2 diabetes. Initial, a solid MedDiet incorporates cell reinforcement luxurious products of the soil, just as fish and nuts; foods that are copious in sound fats. These supplements help support psychological capacity by decreasing irritation and oxidation in the cerebrum.

Furthermore, the MedDiet incorporates entire grains and vegetables that help with keeping glucose at substantial levels. Keeping Type 2 diabetes controlled helps lower metabolic oxidation items and supports proficient insulin activity, which assumes a job in psychological procedures. In this way, the diet may have double benefits on comprehension and glucose control. Both sticking to a Mediterranean diet and adequately overseeing Type 2 diabetes may bolster ideal subjective capacity, the researchers wrote in their decision. Solid foods, when all is said in done, can help improve memory work among grown-ups without Type 2 diabetes.

Exercises to Do with The Mediterranean Diet

It's nothing unexpected that researchers discovered medical advantages from the Mediterranean-style diet, which is overwhelming in lean meats and fish, olive oil, entire grains, vegetables, and products of the soil and low in prepared foods and sugary desserts. Researchers have long realized that the Mediterranean diet seems to ensure against cardiovascular malady. In any case, no one knew precisely why the Mediterranean diet created those advantages. What explicitly does the diet change inside the body that helps heart wellbeing?

Numerous researchers have been on the field, making their discoveries, studies, and different types of probes. Ongoing exploration by a gathering of Nutritionists from Harvard University discovered signs in 25,000 members in the Women's Health Study, looking at the ladies' diets just as 40 distinctive biomarkers. They at that point thought about that data against information on which of the ladies proceeded to have heart assaults, blood vessel blockages, or strokes throughout the around 12-year follow-up period. In addition to the fact that they found that ladies whose diets most intently looked like a customary Mediterranean example were a quarter less inclined to have heart and vein issues than those whose diets least took after that model, they likewise utilized the biomarker data to show signs of improvement picture of precisely what was distinctive about individuals who were eating a Mediterranean-style diet versus the individuals who weren't.

Biomarker information demonstrated that ladies eating a Mediterranean-style diet had upgrades in some significant measures. Contrasted and ladies who didn't eat a Mediterranean-style food, ladies who did saw drops in heart and vein dangers of 29% from a decrease in irritation, which is a known supporter of heart illness 27.9% from improved glucose digestion and a reduction in insulin obstruction 27.3% from lower weight file. Researchers additionally observed enhancements in circulatory strain, cholesterol levels, and different biomarkers, yet these were less huge. Nobody was expecting that the diet would influence every one of these pathways. The drop in interminable irritation seemed to give the most significant level of hazard decrease. It was unexpected that the commitment of irritation was significantly more grounded than the impact on pulse and glucose digestion.

Some accept that the Mediterranean diet may beneficially affect your stomach related tract and the 100 trillion microscopic organisms and different microorganisms that live inside it. Research is uncovering the significance of a diverse and stable intestinal microbiome (the microbial network in the gut), which is presently thought to assume a job in invulnerable capacity and recuperating aggravation inside the body. It's the idea that the Mediterranean-style diet, which incorporates low-sugar Greek yogurt and other aged foods, may contribute sound life forms to the microbiome. A portion of its positive wellbeing impacts may originate from those commitments.

Future research on the diet may likewise take a gander at the job extra-virgin olive oil plays in the dietary advantages of the Mediterranean-style model. Extra-virgin olive oil is accepted to forestall a type of irregular heartbeat known as an arrhythmia, and it's likewise thought to decrease bosom cancer hazard. Other research has uncovered a potential relationship with lower dangers for diabetes and dementia. The more intently ladies pursued the Mediterranean diet, the more upgrades they saw by and large. That doesn't mean you should be impeccable to see medical advantages from dietary changes. Attempt to pursue the Mediterranean diet 80% to 90% of the time, yet you can enable yourself some space to stray — if it remains inside that 10%–20% territory.

Nonetheless, you should stay with the Mediterranean-style design after some time to see a substantial decrease in cardiovascular dangers. This is certifiably not a temporary fix; instead, see it as a way of life change. It should be done reliably. Be that as it may, this investigation demonstrates that leaving on this methodology is probably going to bring substantial advantages. Numerous individuals are bound to change their way of life if they know how it will profit them. "A great deal of us are interested, for what reason would it be a good idea for me to do this? Realizing how something functions are useful.

Fortunately, not at all like some popular craze type diets, the Mediterranean model is generally simple to pursue. The Mediterranean diet is in reality all around endured, and numerous individuals can stick to it over the long haul. Also, it offers a great deal of decision in food choice and doesn't require checking calories. This is a nonrestrictive diet. Indeed, even without calorie tallying, this eating plan could help with weight control. By and large, there was a decrease in weight list among those in the examination who agreed most intimately with the Mediterranean-style diet, yet the progressions were little. Be that as it may, it's critical to take note of that while ladies on a diet didn't see a great deal of weight reduction, the food may have avoided weight gain in certain occurrences, on the grounds that a large number of the Mediterranean-style eaters in the examination kept up their body weight as they entered menopause, when they generally may have picked up.

Researchers at Saint Louis University have discovered that eating a Mediterranean diet can improve competitors' continuance practice execution after only four days. In a little report distributed in the Journal of the American College of Nutrition, agents found that members ran a 5K six percent quicker in the wake of eating a Mediterranean diet than after eating a portion of Western food. Researchers found no contrast between the two diets in execution in anaerobic exercise tests.

The Mediterranean diet incorporates entire products of the soil, nuts, olive oil, and whole grains, and maintains a strategic distance from red and prepared meats, dairy, trans and soaked fats, and refined sugars. By correlation, the Western diet is portrayed by low admission of natural product, vegetables and grungy or negligibly handled oils and high entries of trans and immersed fats, dairy, refined sugars, refined and exceptionally prepared vegetable oils, sodium and processed foods.

The Mediterranean diet is settled as having various medical advantages. It has a great deal of mitigating and cell reinforcement impacts, progressively antacid pH and dietary nitrates which may prompt improved exercise execution. Numerous individual supplements in the Mediterranean diet improve practice execution quickly or inside a couple of days. In this manner, it bodes well that an entire dietary example that incorporates these supplements

75

rushes to improve performance. Notwithstanding, these advantages were likewise rapidly lost when changing toward the Western diet, featuring the significance of long-haul adherence to the Mediterranean diet. The examination selected seven ladies and four men in a randomized-grouping hybrid investigation. The members ran five kilometers on a treadmill on two events—once following four days on a Mediterranean diet and on another event following four days on a Western diet, with a time of nine to 16 days isolating the two tests.

An examination did by a researcher found the 5K run time was six percent quicker after the Mediterranean diet than the Western diet notwithstanding comparative heart rates and evaluations of saw exertion. This study gives proof that a food that is known to be useful for wellbeing is additionally helpful for exercise execution. Like the overall public, competitors and other exercise fans generally eat undesirable diets. Presently they have an extra motivator to practice good eating habits.

Step by step instructions to Lose Weight on a Mediterranean Diet:

You can get in shape on the Mediterranean Diet. Late inquiries about have demonstrated that individuals lost somewhat more weight when following a Mediterranean diet, contrasted with a low-fat diet. They likewise had a minimal increment in midsection periphery contrasted with the low-fat diet. This isn't the first run through the Mediterranean diet has been related with weight reduction, another investigation in 2008 distributed in the New England Journal of Medicine additionally demonstrated that there was more noticeable weight reduction with the Mediterranean diet contrasted with a low-fat diet. Different investigations have additionally connected the Mediterranean diet with a substantial load in kids just as in pregnant ladies.

So, it isn't anything new. Presently, to explain, numerous individuals partner the Mediterranean diet with bunches of pasta and olive oil. That is a misguided judgment, the customary Mediterranean diet that had as a prototype the Cretan food is for the most part plants and olive oil with some carbs mixed, it is a moderate to high-fat diet with a reasonable measure of starches.

If you want to lose weight following a Mediterranean diet here are my 5 tips that work:

1. Eat your primary food promptly in the day time

Customarily inside a Mediterranean diet, lunch is the first meal, it is expended between 1 to 3 pm. By moving a more significant dinner promptly in the day, you decrease the danger of gorging later. Indeed a Spanish report demonstrated that individuals who ate their most significant supper before 3 pm lost more weight.

2. Eat vegetables as a fundamental course cooked in olive oil

This can't be focused on enough, yet this type of dish is the enchantment of the Greek diet. By eating a vegetable dish cooked in olive oil and tomato in addition to the fact that you are fulfilled, you are devouring 3-4 servings of vegetables in a single sitting. These dishes are of moderate caloric level and low in carbs. Go

77

with it with a bit of feta cheddar and you are set. Another advantage of eating vegetables as a first course is that since it's anything but a carb-rich supper, you will maintain a strategic distance from the drowsiness that pursues.

3. You should drink water for the most part and once in a while tea, espresso and wine (for grown-ups)

Indeed, it is standard in individual nations (like the US) to drink milk with dinners, however, is it extremely vital? No. With the Mediterranean diet, most dairy originates from cheddar and yogurt, so spare your calories and use them by eating healthy food as opposed to liquid calories. The equivalent goes for juice. No one needs to squeeze, eat your organic product. They are filling, and you get all the fiber and supplements. Concerning espresso and wine, every ha its place in the Mediterranean diet, however, they don't supplant water. Traditional Greek espresso has been related to a few medical advantages, thus has wine.

4. Expend the perfect measure of olive oil

Increasingly more research is affirming what we here in the Mediterranean know: high fat doesn't make you fat. Truly, calories tally, however, to support a vegetable-based diet, you need something to give satiety and enhance, and that is olive oil. Olive oil not just makes each one of those vegetables flavorful, it makes the dinner filling. That doesn't mean, be that as it may, that you ought to pour olive oil thoughtlessly on everything. A decent sum that is likewise connected with all the medical advantages is around three tablespoons every day.

5. Move

The Mediterranean diet isn't just a diet, it is a way of life, so moving around is basic. Strolling is beautiful, yet broad development for the day is vital. It's insufficient to go to the exercise center for an hour in the first part of the day and afterward sit at your office or on the love seat the remainder of the day. Take strolling breaks, do a few stretches each hour, do housework and on the off chance that you can walk someplace, do that as opposed to driving.

How the Mediterranean Diet Benefits Workout:

You realize that well established saying, "your health will depend on the type of food you eat"? Clearly, so is your exercise. Indeed, when you at first go over any new research proposing that the Mediterranean diet can improve your exercise schedule, you may not be amazed. Many individuals are about a cut of avocado toast, or scooping a tablespoon of nutty spread straight out of the container before hitting the rec center, so it's great to be especially keeping pace with the essential parts that make up the establishment of along these lines of eating as it so happens. Notwithstanding, there's something else entirely to the Mediterranean diet than sound fats and entire grains, and in case you're hoping to support your exhibition run on the track, balling out on the court, or taking laps in the pool, eating Mediterranean-style may be the best approach to do it.

Tune in; many understood that the Mediterranean diet has progressed toward becoming something of a buzz-term around the wellbeing and health space, yet the advantages that this food program brags are nothing to sniffle at. For example, a portion of the medical benefits of a Mediterranean diet incorporates low cholesterol, just as a lower danger of creating heart illness. Likewise? Along these lines of eating may very well enable you to attach a couple of additional years to your life. If that doesn't persuade you to at any rate think about doing the switch, at that point, I don't have a clue what will.

This book isn't tied in with influencing you somehow. If chowing down on a chicken caesar wrap before jumping on the treadmill gets you siphoned, at that point definitely, do you. This book is here to transfer the realities, and as indicated by new inquire about, the truth of the matter is, a Mediterranean diet can improve your continuance practice execution.

These discoveries come as the aftereffect of a little report performed by researchers from Saint Louis University (SLU), who looked at the exhibition of 5K sprinters following a Mediterranean diet to 5K sprinters who pursued a conventional Western diet. Presently, to explain, a Mediterranean diet, for those of you who probably won't know, is involved an abundance of natural products, vegetables, nuts, entire grains, and olive oil. A conventional Western diet is practically the inverse, in that foods grown from the ground bits are low, while handled meats, dairy, prepared sugars, and high soaked fats are the principal center. Realizing that, the consequences of this investigation may not come to all things considered a significant astonishment.

For their investigation, researchers selected seven ladies and four men in their mid-20s and mid-30s, who were told to pursue a Mediterranean or Western diet, per SLU's official statement.

Following four days on each diet, the gathering ran five kilometers on the treadmill. They were then given a nine-to 16-day rest period before changing to the contrary diet for an additional four days, and hustling for a subsequent time. As indicated by the investigation's outcomes, which have been distributed in the Journal of the American College of Nutrition, the individuals who pursued a Mediterranean diet ran 6 percent quicker than those on a Western diet. Since a large number of the individual supplements in the Mediterranean diet have been appeared to "improve practice execution promptly or inside a couple of days," it bodes well that holding fast to the food, in general, would likewise be "speedy to improve execution." However, Weiss included that these advantages were additionally "rapidly lost when changing toward the Western diet, featuring the significance of long haul adherence to the Mediterranean diet."

Along these lines, to explain, as per the American Heart Association, perseverance works out, also called oxygen consuming activity, alludes to "exercises that expansion your breathing and heart rate, for example, strolling, running, swimming, and biking." Anaerobic exercise, per Healthline, is a "higher force, higher power variant of activity," and incorporates practices like bounce restricting, weightlifting, high-force interim preparing (HIIT), and run. Per SLU's public statement, a Mediterranean diet was appeared to help an individual's perseverance practice execution; they found "no distinction between the two diets in execution in anaerobic exercise tests."

Presently, it's critical to know yourself, and it will make you feel more empowered to work out when you have stacked up on

81

leafy foods, and only foods all in all that isn't as substantial on your stomach (ahem, meats and dairy). That distinction in vitality all comes down to the starches you're placing into your body. In this way, instead of empowering you, essential carbs, for example, dairy, prepared loaves of bread, just as foods high in sugars (which are for the most part ordinarily found in a Western diet), really have the contrary impact — for example, they regularly cause you to feel lazy. Complex carbs and lean proteins found in a Mediterranean diet, then again, can offer the vitality you have to support quality execution all through your exercises.

Things being what they are, would it be advisable for you to jump on the Mediterranean train? It indeed relies upon your objectives. As usual, however, make a point to check in with your primary care physician before rolling out any vast improvements to your diet, since what's appropriate for these competitors may not bode well for your body (however, a couple of new greens to a great extent surely can't hurt).

Specialists, much of the time, advises large patients, especially those with a metabolic disorder, to get more fit by embracing a reliable way of life. While low-fat and low-carb diets help temporarily, investigate doesn't bolster their extended haul benefits. Another examination found the blend of the Mediterranean diet (MedDiet) and exercise advanced weight reduction and decreased cardiovascular hazard, benefits that were kept up following one year.

In the examination distributed in the diary Diabetes Care, researchers contemplated 626 overweight patients between the ages of 55 and 75. The members had in any event three of the accompanying cardiovascular hazard factors: hypertension, stomach heftiness, high blood sugar levels, low HDL cholesterol, and high triglycerides. Researchers observed changes in fat gathering, body weight, and a variety of cardiovascular hazard markers all through a year. The outcomes demonstrated that utilization of the MedDiet, which is usually low in calories, prompted, at any rate, a five-percent weight decrease. What's more, the members experienced enhancements in provocative markers and glucose digestion contrasted with the individuals who didn't pursue the diet — also, patients who had diabetics or danger of diabetes delighted in particularly high glucose control benefits.

As per the exploration group, the most weight reduction was noted following a year, a finding that demonstrates the weight decrease was kept up after some time. They reasoned that the MedDiet and a customary exercise program might deliver long haul favorable circumstances for cardiovascular illness, which would convert into fewer passings from heart assaults and strokes.

Craze diets like low-carb diets enable individuals to shed pounds rapidly, yet we have to take a gander at their maintainability and their effect on long haul wellbeing. Such foods are challenging to pursue over an extensive stretch, and they convey cardiovascular dangers. This is the reason to lean toward the MedDiet, which can be utilized from the extremely youthful to the old. It's the perfect eating design since it advances weight the board, alongside numerous different health benefits.

The MedDiet has been investigated broadly. Studies show it decreases the probability of cardiovascular sickness, Alzheimer's infection, blood clumps, and metabolic disorder. The proof additionally demonstrates the diet improves insulin affectability, brings down oxidative pressure, diminishes irritation, and upgrades endothelial cell work. Utilization of the dangerous American food, which is calorie-thick, supplement drained and exceptionally handled, prompts numerous medicinal issues. On the other hand, the natural foods that contain the MedDiet furnish the body with supplements it needs to amplify wellbeing. It's wealthy in organic products, vegetables, vegetables, fatty fish, nuts, seeds, and additional virgin olive oil. The eating plan is likewise low in red meat and sugary drinks.

Consolidating the MedDiet with exercise can do a lot to avert ailment. As I said as of late at the Obesity Medicine Association Fall Conference, patients can regularly accomplish more with a blade and fork and great pair of strolling shoes to keep up ideal wellbeing than we can do with prescriptions, stents, and surgical tools. The Mediterranean diet offers a scope of advantages, from cardioprotective impacts to fighting off interminable illness. Therefore, researchers are progressively calling attention to that this diet might be the way into long, sound life. The Mediterranean diet — which is commonly wealthy in natural products, vegetables, entire grains, nuts, seeds, and olive oil, and permits moderate utilization of fish, dairy, and red wine — contains different aggravates that athletic lift execution. A large number of the foods in the Mediterranean diet contain cell reinforcements and nitrates and have calming and alkalizing properties. Things being what they are, does this imply by adhering to this diet, an individual will experience improved perseverance and exercise execution?

A gathering of researchers enlisted seven ladies and four men who were "recreationally dynamic." After four days of following the prevalently plant-based diet, the researchers requested that the members run 5 kilometers (km) on a treadmill. Nine to 16 days after the fact, the researchers asked that similar members pursue a Western diet for an additional four days and take the 5 km treadmill test once more. A Western diet is ordinarily described by an over-utilization and decreased the assortment of refined sugars, salt, and soaked fat.

The researchers likewise needed to test the impacts that these two diets would have on anaerobic or muscle-fortifying activity. Along these lines, they requested that the members take a cycle test, a vertical hop test, and a handgrip test simultaneously focuses all through the investigation. Generally speaking, the research found that individuals were 6 percent quicker in the 5 km treadmill pursue following the Mediterranean diet than they were after holding fast to a Western diet.

This improvement happened even though the members' heart rates were about the equivalent, and they felt similarly as worn out on the two events. Paradoxically, the diets didn't have any impact on execution in anaerobic exercise. Prof. Weiss and partners close: Our discoveries expand the existing proof of the medical advantages of the Mediterranean diet by demonstrating that this diet is additionally successful for improving continuance practice execution in as meager as four days. Numerous individual supplements in the Mediterranean diet improve practice execution promptly or inside a couple of days. In this manner, it bodes well that an entire dietary example that incorporates these supplements rushes to improve execution. In any case, these advantages were likewise rapidly lost when changing toward the Western diet, featuring the significance of long-haul adherence to the Mediterranean diet," the creator reports.

This examination gives proof that a diet that is known to be useful for wellbeing is additionally helpful for exercise execution. Like the overall public, competitors and other exercise fans regularly eat unhealthy foods. Presently they have an extra impetus to eat [healthfully].

A Mediterranean diet and legitimate exercise may prompt longer life expectancies among the clinically stout, as per another examination. Researchers from the Montreal Heart Institute (MIH) in Canada have established that high-force interim preparing joined with a diet wealthy in beans, nuts, grains, and vegetables may bring about a critical decrease in the cardiovascular wellbeing dangers related with stomach stoutness. The discoveries add to the developing assemblage of proof that a sound heart is a way into a more drawn out life.

The investigation, which was reported at the Canadian Cardiovascular Congress, tried to assess how a Mediterranean diet and physical exercise impact the run of the mill hazard elements going to a weight record (BMI) surpassing 30. While both wellness and dieting have been investigated autonomously in comparable limits before, the new examination inspected whether a mix of the two would expand their medical advantages.

Every one of this way of life mediations alone is known to affect; however, nobody has examined them together in a more extended term," he said in a public statement. Our outcomes demonstrate that the blend of the two mediations supersized the advantages to heart wellbeing.

To evaluate the advantages of a Mediterranean diet in the mix with interim preparing, the researchers enlisted a gathering of abdominally corpulent individuals in an investigation. The members experienced high-force interim preparing a few times each week while accepting ceaseless dietary advising. After nine months, the regular member showed noteworthy outcomes.

As per the researchers, improved cardiovascular wellness leads to a whole range of medical advantages, incorporating decreases in midriff boundary, cholesterol, blood weight, weight, and BMI. Furthermore, the members demonstrated an emotional improvement in muscle continuance and exercise limit. "What is striking isn't just the positive early outcomes, which can be healthy when inspiration is high, yet the way that members continued improving into a subsequent year.

The Mediterranean diet has been attached to various medical advantages in past food examine. As per the Mayo Clinic, the food depends on the organic product, vegetables, beans, vegetables, and nuts as the establishment of each supper. Furthermore, the diet stresses:

- Eating primarily plant-based foods, for example, foods grown from the ground, entire grains, vegetables and nuts

- Supplanting margarine with sound fats, for example, olive oil

- Utilizing herbs and flavors rather than salt to season foods

87

- Restricting red meat to close to a couple of times each month

- Eating fish and poultry, at any rate, two times per week

- Reasons You Are Not Losing Weight on the Mediterranean Diet

The Mediterranean diet has picked up ubiquity as an excellent method to get thinner and improve wellbeing. Its supporters eating more plant-based foods like natural products, vegetables, nuts, vegetables, just as eating fish and poultry, in any event, two times every week. The diet additionally includes swapping out margarine for olive or canola oil, getting a charge out of suppers with others, and enhancing food with herbs and flavors rather than salt.

Eating this way has been related to a lower danger of heart sickness and the bringing down of "awful" LDL cholesterol. The Mediterranean diet has additionally been connected to decreased frequency of cancer, and Parkinson's and Alzheimer's diseases. What's more, even though the Mediterranean diet is known to have a large group of medical advantages, including weight reduction, a few people may find that they're not losing much weight even while adhering to the diet.

Nutritionists, dietitians, and specialists were counseled to make sense of why you probably won't shed pounds on the Mediterranean diet.

- You're adding an excessive amount of olive oil to your suppers

The Mediterranean diet supports the utilization of solid fats like additional virgin olive oil and other monounsaturated fats instead of immersed fats, for example, spread and grease. In any case, the way to making these swaps work for weight reduction is giving close consideration to how much fat you're utilizing.

Olive oil (and all oils) give 120 calories and 14 grams of fat for each tablespoon. Since numerous individuals utilize substantially more than that, several abundance calories are expended. Even though a teaspoon or tablespoon of additional virgin olive oil will add flavor and supplements to your dish, broiling vegetables with a quarter cup of the stuff can likewise add many unnecessary calories to your feast.

When preparing your decent feast, don't go over the edge adding additional olive oil to your food. Limited quantities still give benefits; however, they can keep the calories in your supper low.

- You're eating an excessive number of nuts without acknowledging it

Nuts are an extraordinary plant-based tidbit – they're convenient, delicious, and pack a hit of protein. They're additionally a heavenly wellspring of the omega-3 ALA and a vibrant vitality part of Mediterranean diets. Be that as it may, numerous individuals genuinely think little of the number of calories they're expending when they eat nuts.

One-quarter cup of nuts ordinarily contains 150 to 200 calories. Numerous individuals think that it's effortless to nibble on more

89

than 1,000 calories of nuts in a sitting, so it is critical to be aware of part measures with the goal that you don't attack yourself.

- You're drinking an excessive amount of red wine or liquor

For some individuals, one of the top-selling purposes of the Mediterranean diet is the consideration of red wine. It's not essential to drink wine to be agreeable with the Mediterranean diet; however, any individual who does so needs to consider the calories in that wine. On the off chance that you are inexperienced with the subtleties of this diet, it's anything but difficult to over-expend calories from liquor and consequently disrupting weight reduction endeavors. A serving of wine is just 5 ounces, and balance means up to one glass for every day for ladies and two drinks for each day for men.

To be certain beyond a shadow of a doubt, you're not fixing your diet with a substantial pour of wine, set aside the effort to quantify how much wine you're expending and adhere to the suggested day by day limit for your body type.

- You're not considering other fluid calories

Regardless of whether you're cautious about constraining the measure of red wine, you drink on the Mediterranean diet, not watching out for your other fluid calories could be undermining your diet. Individuals consider food as far as substantial food, yet 40% of our calories can emerge out of beverages. On the off chance that we have such a large number of sweet mixed drinks, Frappuccinos, or as far as anyone knows to sound organic product juices, individuals don't think they are breaking their diet, yet they could add to calories fundamentally.

Because something is advertised as being "sound" doesn't mean it won't influence your waistline. Make certain to peruse the wholesome marks on all your pre-made beverages and decide on entire products of the soil over smoothies and juices when conceivable.

- You're not controlling part measures

The Mediterranean diet incorporates a lot of wellbeing advancing foods as it is as yet conceivable to put on weight in case, you're eating a more significant number of calories than you're consuming. The Mediterranean diet is a brilliantly sound approach to eat, yet individuals can devour an excessive number of calories on practically any food. Best weight reduction diets adjust both the type of food eaten just as the sum. In case you're not doing both, you likely won't get in shape.

Heaping your plate high with diet-accommodating foods can ruin your weight reduction endeavors in case you're not focusing on bit size. Fortunately, you don't require a scale to make sense of the amount to eat on this diet as you parcel your Mediterranean-style plate, attempt to make half of it vegetables with high water substance, for example, zucchini, eggplant, onion, and peppers. Cutoff the grain choice to only one-fourth of your feast. Keep the protein decision to a sum the size of your palm.

- You depend on "solid" swaps without thinking about calories

There's no chance to get around it: when you're attempting to get more fit, calories matter. The diet urges adherents to swap out processed foods and sugary treats for organic products, veggies, fish, and healthy fats. However, it's as yet critical to monitor what number of calories you're expending. Calorie-stacked foods that have a youthful radiance like avocado, nuts and intemperate measures of olive oil are incredibly caloric thick and can pack fat rapidly on your waistline.

Entire grains like entire wheat flour, darker rice, bulgur, and grain are staples in the Mediterranean diet, however basically swapping out white flour and rice for dark-colored assortments won't spare calories. Basically, swapping entire wheat flour for white flour doesn't naturally mean solid. For instance, your entire grain biscuit can at present be larger than average, giving more than 600 calories and contain unfortunate fixings.

- You're not including calories from garnishes and sauces

Regardless of whether you've remembered the number of calories in a sweet potato and have splendidly partitioned your pasta, garnishes and sauces can add surprising calories to a feast. Your diet isn't as clean and low in calories as you might suspect. The shrouded saboteurs are all over, from an excessive amount of serving of mixed greens dressing to espresso half and half. There are a thousand easily overlooked details that can pack on many calories.

- You're overestimating what number of calories you're consuming

Except if you go through your day doing physical work or are a functioning competitor, you likely won't shed pounds eating 2,000 calories for each day except if you're fusing exercise into your everyday practice. Primarily, just strolling up a couple of flights of stairs to arrive at your office won't consume enough calories to qualify as an exercise. Numerous individuals overestimate the calories they consume in a day overall by as much as 25%. Follow along and utilize a diary or an application.

- You're concentrating on diet and overlooking the activity

The Mediterranean diet is about something beyond your staple rundown. To receive the weight reduction rewards of this way of eating, you can't disregard the remaining dynamic. Even though it is conceivable to get thinner by altering diet alone, it is troublesome. Adding customary exercise to any weight reduction routine builds your odds of consuming a more significant number of calories than you expend, causing you to shed pounds all the more reliably.

All weight reduction plans profits by a guarantee to exercise and consuming calories. To make the Mediterranean a viable weight reduction system, make sure to keep your body moving.

- You're eating too rapidly and not relishing your food

The Mediterranean diet advances a style of eating that goes past what's on your plate. Making this diet work means grasping that suppers are about something other than calories and supplements. Make the most of your food by setting aside the effort to look for new fixings, invest energy cooking with companions or family, and wait at the table.

Don't merely embrace the foods from a Mediterranean plan, accept this open the door to developing their frame of mind towards eating, as well. When you center around easing back your speed of eating down, you're probably going to feel progressively fulfilled on less food. To ensure you're not trying too hard, predivide your nuts in plastic packs or reusable compartments to ensure you can appreciate the medical advantages without unintentionally eating more than you intended to.

- You're pushed

Even though diet and exercise are vital bits of the weight reduction baffle, researchers are beginning to comprehend that our feelings of anxiety can influence the amount we weigh — individuals who live with long haul pressure experience great introduction to the hormone cortisol. High cortisol can build insulin discharge and your ability to store sugars as fat.

On the off chance that following the Mediterranean diet isn't helping you with your weight reduction venture, it may merit investigating pressure decrease systems like contemplation or yoga. Conversing with an analyst or authorized specialist can likewise help settle any severe subject matters that might hinder your weight reduction endeavors.

- You're not getting enough rest

So, you've supplied your kitchen with sound foods and are adhering to the Mediterranean diet at each dinner. Be that as it may, in case you're not getting enough rest during the evening, you could, in any case, be incidentally defeating your weight reduction endeavors.

Frequently individuals who are focused on additionally experience rest interruption as well, which is likewise connected to an expanded danger of overweight and heftiness because of its capacity to upset hormones that direct completion and craving. Watching your preferred shows late into the night may be without calorie. But remember, the subsequent lack of sleep could be undermining the positive changes you've made to your diet. Make sure to get around eight hours of value rest every night to help bolster your weight reduction objectives.

Lifestyle Lessons to Emulate with the Mediterranean Diet

Hear this stunning story from somebody who is from the Mediterranean region. It's only a short story of a way of life that can be copied to make simple. You can pick a few points from it while carrying on with the life of the Mediterranean Diet.

"I was one of those individuals who did everything right growing up. I considered, got decent evaluations, showed signs of improvement employments, and kept out of the issue. I never needed to frustrate my outsider guardians, who had relinquished and rationed with the goal that my kin and I could move on from school obligation-free.

95

Whenever companions and flat mates were traipsing crosswise over Europe, running with the bulls in Pamplona, connecting with Greek divine beings at open-air discos, or trekking the Great Wall, I worked and contemplated. I spent school summers working in a grassroots association, a political campaigning gathering, or as an understudy at the Virginia General Assembly.

One summer in school, I verified a temporary position on a remote island in the Mediterranean. That mid-year in Cyprus transformed me. I came back to the University of Virginia stricken with this old island, the flawless locals, and their casual, sound way of life. It didn't hurt that I was likewise hit with a person. I didn't have any acquaintance with it at the time, yet I had met my future spouse.

A long-time later, this running youthful Cypriot and I wedded. We lived in Atlanta, where I had earned a useful MBA in money and a lucrative, however (for me) sub-par corporate presence.

I went through hours out and about or fastened to my work area. Even though our bankroll developed and we had two lovely youngsters, I felt something was missing. That far off summer in Cyprus was an ever-present token of how life ought to be: more beneficial, progressively loose, and increasingly adjusted among work and play.

With two children close behind, my better half and I chose to pack up our Atlanta home and move east to Cyprus for what was initially planned to be just for a couple of pf years. Be that as it may, life dominated; we got dependent on the Mediterranean sun and stayed on the island of Aphrodite.

Throughout the years, I took in some things about how to unwind, relish life, and live like a Mediterranean goddess."

- My cabinets are uncovered, yet my ice chest is full.

In my corporate days, secured ten or more hours a work area or making a trip to various urban communities week by week, I munched on granola bars, tasted on Diet Coke, and nibbled on dry Fruity Pebbles late around evening time.

Handled foods usurp our American staple walkways. On the island, we eat three appropriate suppers. Tidbits are entire natural product or nuts.

Today my dinners are focused round occasional, privately developed products of the soil. Sauces, treats, and wafers (on the off chance that they exist in my kitchen) are little boxes and appreciated sparingly (bye, bye Costco-size!).

- Everyone eats fat, yet nobody gets fat

I used to fixate on eating low-fat pretzels, low-fat biscuits, low-fat yogurt, and so forth. In the Mediterranean, full-fat yogurt and milk, sheep, fatty fish, nuts, olive oil, and entire grains include our diets.

It's considered far superior (and increasingly scrumptious) to relish a half-cup of full-fat yogurt than to eat a compartment of flavorless nonfat yogurt, improved with syrup and phony organic product.

97

- I skirted the exercise center and began a nursery

I cherished my old training camp classes, yet without an ex-Marine shouting his head off at overweight, overprivileged office laborers, I figured out how to go for long strolls through the slopes or somewhere near the beach with my family and canine.

Working my very own territory; planting cilantro, cucumbers, and tomatoes, weeding, and watering until the natural product developed ready: This is one of the primary manners by which Mediterranean individuals live invigoratingly — less pressure, additionally residing outside.

- Adopt a giving nature

I experienced childhood in Virginia, so I intend no lack of respect to the thought of Southern neighborliness, yet there is no correlation with Mediterranean friendliness. We as a whole love getting stuff—unconditional presents, swag sacks, birthday or Christmas presents. It is continuously amusing to get. In the Mediterranean, there is a desire to give consistently. So, if the vast majority are offering, at that point a great many people are likewise accepting. It's a goliath hover of being decent.

We appear at somebody's home with a container of wine, a few cuts of handcrafted cake, or organic product from the nursery. Whatever is close by, a straightforward token of much gratitude goes far.

Also, if you don't have anything to give, a grin and a compliment will light up anybody's day.

- I quit being a handyman and stayed with (and benefit from) a solitary one.

I examined business. I should know my center qualities. Should. Through my 20s, I bounced starting with one occupation then onto the next, with the reason that I was making vertical hops. In truth, I experienced considerable difficulties settling down and creating center capabilities.

Although I earned an accounting degree, my regular tendency was in expressions of the human experience. I examined show, theater, and screenwriting. These specialized aptitudes were what enabled me to, in the long run, take a risk and work for myself.

In Cyprus, my American pronunciation was sought after. I had my radio show and worked intensely on TV. In the end, I propelled a kids' venue school, encouraging neighborhood and expat kids the adoration for dramatization.

Primary concern: Find out what fulfills you. Pick an exchange and profit from it.

- Learn the language—or if nothing else some decision phrases

Americans are happy individuals. We accept we have the best country on the planet. Be that as it may, prepare to have your mind blown. Numerous other individuals feel a similar path about their nation.

In less than two years, I could communicate in the neighborhood language. Expats wondered about how I had gotten the word so rapidly. (Turkish isn't an instinctive language to learn as a local English speaker.)

In any case, prepare to have your mind blown. Local people cherished it! Albeit English is generally spoken all over this beautiful planet, don't be the inconsiderate explorer. Get familiar with their language, their traditions, and their way of life. We are visitors in their nation."

- The world is littler than you might suspect.

When we lived in Atlanta, my significant other and I had precisely three guests: an old companion from New York City who descended for a young ladies' end of the week and my folks the week after my little girl was conceived.

For some odd reason (note: This is a mockery), living on a Mediterranean island inspired loved ones from distant locations abroad to visit. They appeared in the wonder of our capacity to pack up and move over the world.

High school, and graduate school companions; far off cousins; kin; and all the more all came by the thousand to visit. We even had a love bird couple spend some portion of their wedding trip with us. Correspondence and innovation have been a raft for me. Stay aware of your old companions! No one can tell who may require a hand or a pad to lay their head on for a couple of evenings.

How to Set Your Goals for Weight Loss:

Working out, eating more beneficial, and timing more extended periods of rest are for the most part objectives you may set when you need to shed a couple of pounds. Be that as it may, you're human, and the general aim of eating more beneficial may appear to be entirely unclear when you've had an unpleasant day, and you detect some pizza or doughnuts in the gathering room.

Enter the smaller than usual objective, or the little objective, or anything you desire to call them. These small-scale benchmarks may enable you to accomplish significant weight reduction without a tremendous amount of exertion. Are you intrigued? Here, we've gathered together some subtle inspirational methods to allow you to keep your eyes on the thin down prize.

- Aim High

In a recent report, 46 ladies who anticipated they'd shed more weight over a 27-week diet period dropped more pounds (37 all things considered) than those with less grandiose targets (they lost as meager as 13). These difficulties the regular conviction that defining higher-arriving at objectives could make dieters desert transport. The discoveries may move another weight reduction methodology: Set a goal-oriented enormous picture objective, at that point, celebrate at littler gradual focuses. I will propose losing up to 10 percent of your weight in a half year as an objective. You'll gain ground toward your real purpose, yet your prosperity en route will give progressing inspiration.

- Sign Up for Fitness Events

101

A 5K, a mud run, whatever—in case you're attempting to make wellness part of your long-haul weight-reduction plan, including little rivalries en route can enable you to stay aware of your exercise routine. How about we be genuine, hopping on the treadmill sounds much all the more tempting when you realize a race is approaching in your future.

- Add More Spices to Your Meals

I adore the straightforward, little objective of adding more flavors to your diet to support sustenance without expanding calories. There is an abundance of research on the medical advantages of characters, and they can enable your body to oversee insulin better, which can allow you to arrive at your weight reduction objectives. Have a go at adding cinnamon to your cereal or turmeric to your smoothie.

- Eat a Lot of Veggies

No compelling reason to patch up your entire diet—adding more shading to your plate is a simple objective to set. Eating more veggies will expand your fiber admission, keeping you fuller, so you won't be enticed to gorge or bite. Mean to fill at any rate half of your plate with the vivid stuff.

- Take a Lot of Walks

There is enormous research on the negative wellbeing impacts of sitting excessively, regardless of whether you work out. Furthermore, since each carbohydrate content, discovering more approaches to add steps to your day can enable you to lose more weight. Start by setting an update on your calorie to get up and move, strolling to places you would regularly drive, or rising right on time to pile on specific means before anything else. At that point, expect to expand your separation or steps every week.

Planning Weight Loss Goals:

Defining weight reduction objectives is presumably one of the more troublesome strides of a health improvement plan. What amount do you have to lose, and how would you compute that number? The route the vast majority of us approach it is to pick a number dependent on what we used to gauge or, maybe, what we've for a long while been itching to gauge. In any case, is that a sensible objective?

In case you're getting more fit for your wellbeing, your objective may be increasingly unassuming, express 5 to 10 percent of your present weight. Be that as it may, imagine a scenario where you have something progressively explicit as a top priority like a specific attire size you need to fit into. The issue is, there isn't generally a set weight that compares to dress size and, for ladies, apparel sizes vary from organization to organization. All in all, what's the response to these inquiries? Your initial step is to figure out how to set reachable weight reduction objectives that you can quantify.

The way to defining weight reduction objectives is to keep the standard of objective setting, which means it should be SMART. A savvy purpose is: Specific, quantifiable, feasible, reasonable, and unmistakable.

Go right straightforward and start by making sense of on the off chance that you genuinely need to get in shape.

Getting more fit, is it truly required?

On the off chance that you converse with the vast majority, you'll presumably find that everybody feels like they have to get thinner, even individuals who seem, by all accounts, to be at a substantial weight.

Frequently our weight reduction objectives depend on what we figure we ought to resemble as opposed to what's sensible for our bodies at this moment. There are expansive parameters to use to make sense of on the off chance that you have to get more fit in any case, all in all, a possibility for weight reduction may have the accompanying qualities:

- A BMI of more than 25.

- A midriff hip proportion of higher than .8 for ladies and higher than 1.0 men.

- A stomach bigness estimation of more than 35 creeps in ladies and 40 crawls in men.

Those aren't the main pieces of information that reveal to us we have to get in shape. There are those irritating signs like tight garments, escaping breath doing straightforward exercises, or stepping on a scale without precedent for some time. In any case, before you set objectives dependent on what you figure, you ought to gauge, converse with your PCP. The individual will, for the most part, approach tallness weight graphs or different assets that can enable you to make sense of a substantial weight territory for your body type.

Having a Good Weight Loss Goal Setting Plan: If you've decided you do need to get in shape, your subsequent stage is to set a sensible weight reduction objective for yourself. You can put together your objectives concerning any number of elements, yet an excellent spot to begin would be the general suggestions set out by the American College of Sports Medicine which are 5-10% of body weight or one to two pounds for every week. This weight reduction number cruncher will enable you to set an everyday calorie focus to accomplish your weight reduction objectives best. Your outcomes will allow you to concentrate less on actual weight and more on settling on reliable decisions every day to diminish your calories.

The day by day calorie objective from the mini-computer above is the number of calories you ought to eat each day to arrive at your ideal load in the period you set. This made your calorie shortage (with diet and exercise) and your body will react to that after some time. In the end, you'll get to a weight you can support and like.

Have Your Plan: However, you decide your weight reduction objectives, you should record that objective and after that make an arrangement to arrive at it. Take a gander at your target impartially: is it explicit, quantifiable, feasible, reasonable, and unmistakable?

Here's an example of perceiving how it functions:

105

Mary is 5'7" tall and gauges 160 pounds. Her BMI is 25.1, which falls into the 'overweight' classification. On the off chance that she shed only 10 pounds; her BMI would be more beneficial at 23.5. Mary will probably shed 10 pounds in 12 weeks. To do that she would need to slice or exercise off 300 to 500 calories every day. Utilizing a blend of diet and exercise is the ideal approach to shed pounds since dieting alone can make you lose bulk.

Bulk is more metabolically dynamic than fat5, so you need to keep all the muscle you have and include more with quality preparing.

Mary's plan to contact her objectives:
- Replace her morning Egg McMuffin (300 calories) with a bowl of oats (around 180 calories).

- Replace one Coke (150 calories) with shining water (0 calories).

- Walk for in any event 30 minutes at 3.5-4.0 mph, three days every week (approx. 180-240 calories consumed).

- Strength train two days per week for 30 minutes (approx. 140-280 calories consumed)

With this plan, she will consume an aggregate of 270-550 calories every day (contingent upon whether she works out).

Taking a gander at this model, you can see that these are genuinely modest changes. Mary isn't patching up her whole diet; she's essentially picking a couple of things she can change to begin. Exciting that, as she proceeds with her sound practices, she'll start to do much more since she needs to get in shape as well as because she's going to begin feeling good, more grounded, increasingly confident.

Have a go at separating your objective into explicit advances this way and keep tabs on your development. Make sure to change your aim at whatever point you have to. On the off chance that you find you're not shedding pounds as fast as you suspected (and this is exceptionally ordinary), change your actual weight or the period to arrive at it. Keep in mind; your objective should be feasible, so be happy to set new goals if the old ones aren't working for you.

How to Lose Weight on the Mediterranean Diet

Weight reduction is a significant issue for some individuals (and maybe you) on the planet today. You might search for an approach to lose some weight and imagine that the Mediterranean diet is the best approach. Picking a Mediterranean diet won't be a conventional "diet" or a convenient solution. Or maybe, it's a progression of a reliable way of life decisions that can get you to your weight reduction objective while you eat delightful, tasty foods and get out and appreciate life. Sounds much superior to checking calories and denying yourself, isn't that so?

In light of that depiction, you have to concentrate on a couple of absolute necessities with the Mediterranean way of life to get in shape effectively. You need to focus on a way of life changes, deal with your calorie admission through adjusting food decisions and controlling segments, and increment your physical action.

107

- Focus on a Change on General Lifestyle

The focal point of the Mediterranean diet is on your whole way of life. Focusing on a way of life changes, for example, changing your segment sizes and practicing consistently, is the best way to see long haul results. Weight reduction diets travel every which way, and most can enable you to lose the weight, yet they aren't something you can live with the long haul.

The Mediterranean diet encourages you to focus on your way of life, including the sorts of foods you eat, the bit sizes you expend, your physical exercises, and your general lifestyle. You can fuse these progressions into your day by day life and make long haul propensities that bring you weight reduction as well as sustained weight reduction.

- Consume More Calories

Calories are one of the most essential ideas of weight reduction. Fundamentally, calories are the measure of vitality in the foods you eat, and the standard of energy your body utilizes for everyday exercises. Your body continually needs vitality or fuel not just for day by day exercises, for example, cooking, cleaning, and practicing yet additionally for fundamental organic capacities (like, you know, relaxing). Everybody has an alternate metabolic rate that decides how rapidly the individual in question consumes calories and relies upon variables, for example, age, hereditary qualities, sexual orientation, and physical wellness level. Toward the day's end, you can't get thinner if you eat a more significant number of calories than you consume everyday action and exercise. To get leaner, you need to make a calorie shortfall, yet you can do as such without really knowing what number of calories you consume. You should roll out little improvements to your way of life, for example, diminishing segment sizes and practicing more, to decrease your calorie admission. To stay aware of the utilization of more calories, these things ought to be placed into full practice to accomplish the ideal weight reduction system:

- Eat more to get in shape

Dissimilar to many weight reduction diets, a Mediterranean style of eating gives you a chance to have more food on your plate while as yet taking in fewer calories. Eat unquestionably increasingly low-calorie vegetables and less unhealthy meats and grains. To sweeten the deal even further, these lower-calorie foods additionally help you feel progressively happy with your supper as opposed to feeling denied.

- Take bit size into record

Focusing on segment sizes is a much better approach to diminish your calorie admission than checking calories. Segment estimates in the Mediterranean are not the same as they are in the United States, which is one explanation people in the Mediterranean district will in general deal with their loads all the more adequately.

- Watch your fat calories

The Mediterranean diet likewise enables you to monitor the calories you get from fat. Even though individuals on the Mediterranean coast eat somewhat more fat than is suggested in the United States (35 percent of their calories originate from fat, versus the U.S. proposal of 30 percent), they devour various sorts of fat, for example, the solid fats from olive oil.

- Increase the movement you adore.

Exercise is a significant part to weight reduction and wellbeing, particularly with the Mediterranean diet. You need to go through a portion of your calorie consumption as vitality, or those calories will store as fat. Exercise enables you to consume calories as well as fortify your heart, oversee pressure, and increment your vitality level.

- Suppress your hunger

Eating a Mediterranean style diet isn't incredible for your wellbeing however can likewise fill in as a characteristic craving suppressant to help deal with your weight. When you eat the correct equalization of plant-based foods and solid fats, your body works in a particular manner to feel fulfilled. Since you're full, you're not enticed (in any event, not by your stomach) to nibble on unhealthy shoddy food a brief time after your last supper.

The Mediterranean diet is ordinarily high in low-glycemic foods, those starch-containing food sources that unlawful a lower glucose spike. Low-glycemic foods may help kick on your completion reaction. Craving is constrained by a multifaceted move of hormones that trigger the sentiments of appetite and completion.

- Control food yearnings

Food yearnings happen for some reasons, regardless of whether they're physiological, mental, or a blend of both. For example, having an upsetting day at work may prompt food longings. Shockingly, nobody size-fits-all-answer exists to manage food longings but you can do a couple of things to oversee them all the more viably. Put these things as the main priority as well:

- Make sure you don't skip suppers or stand by longer than 5 hours to eat. Eat a feast or nibble each 3 to 5 hours. Eat when you are ravenous as opposed to holding up until you have an extraordinary craving.

- Eat protein-rich food and a touch of fat. Incorporate foods, for example, fish, beans, nuts, or eggs with fat with every supper to help hinder your processing.

- Eat high-fiber, organic products, vegetables, grains, and vegetables with every feast and bite. You don't need to eat these foods at the same time, however, including a blend of them at dinners and joining an organic product, veggie, or entire grain with your tidbits is a smart thought.

- Manage your pressure hormones: You can achieve this by working out, getting enough rest, drinking water, rehearsing profound breathing, contemplating, and unwinding. For instance, on the off chance that you are preparing for an unpleasant gathering, take a couple of minutes to do some profound relaxing. Take a full breath, hold it for a couple of moments, and let them freshen up. Continue rehashing for whatever length of time that you can. Indeed, even a couple of minutes can help.

111

A Lifestyle for Good Health and Weight Management

May is the Mediterranean Diet Month, an opportunity to appraise the food conventions of the countries encompassing the Mediterranean Sea, including Italy, Spain, Greece, Turkey, and Morocco.

Touted as probably the most advantageous methods for eating, it's simple, spending plan agreeable, and well, indeed less a diet (as in, "I'm on a diet"), as a way of life. In this way, on the off chance that it truly isn't a diet really, you may think about whether it's workable for individuals to shed pounds when they tail it. For some individuals, they can.

The Mediterranean diet is tied in with eating an equalization of leafy foods, lean meats, for example, chicken and fish, entire grains, vegetables and beans, nuts, seeds, dairy, eggs, olives, and olive oil, you'll have a lot of nutritious and scrumptious decisions to put on your plate. The key is to eat a parity of these foods and appreciate them with some restraint. Studies have over and again confirmed the wellbeing benefits of this way of eating, including being more effective than a low-fat diet with regards to weight reduction.

In opposition to prevalent thinking, eating admirably can be affordable. The Mediterranean Diet way of life can be spending agreeable on the off chance that you pick produce that is in season and privately developed, it's supplement thick and eases. On the off chance that purchasing new isn't a choice or if you need to change up your diet, pick solidified or canned veggies and organic product which is similarly nutritious and efficient. Solidified and canned things are ideal for keeping in your washroom as they're always prepared for a minute ago supper thoughts or extending your food spending plan. Make sure to search for things that are low in sodium with no additional sugars.

Notwithstanding the luscious foods of this locale, different parts of thusly of life incorporate getting a charge out of the delights of the table with family and companions, remaining physically dynamic every day, (for example, an after-supper walk or taking the stairs at whatever point conceivable), picking entire food sources over-prepared, and cooking dinners at home. As you appreciate the flavorful foods of the Mediterranean Diet, these practical tips can enable you to remain on track with your weight reduction objectives:

- Know what you're eating. When purchasing prepared foods, read the fixing rundown and Nutrition Facts board to see precisely what's in your food, the calories, and serving size. I propose that you utilize the Daily Value and the 5/20 guideline for a brisk and straightforward approach to peruse the mark. Five percent is viewed as low, and 20% is considered to be high. Recognizing foods with significant levels (at any rate 20% DV) of healthy vitamins and supplements and low levels (under 5% DV) of sodium, soaked fats, and sugars will enable you to know which food sources to go after frequently.

- Don't skip dinners, doing so can make you eager and progressively inclined to attacking the refrigerator or candy machine.

113

- Cook and appreciate more dinners at home. You'll likely spare calories just as an admission of fat, sugar, and sodium when you control the fixings.

- It is likewise energized that participating in careful eating by appreciating each nibble of food and the discussion of family and companions, which can enable us to feel fuller with less food.

- Cook once. Eat twice. When planning family meals, remember lunch. For instance, when simmering a chicken, making an entire grain or pasta dish, or making soup or stew, make extra for lunch. It's conservative and enables slice food to squander, as well.

- Another tip to pursue as you put together your lunch for the day is to remember sanitation. Incorporate an ice pack to keep your fresh foods cold and a protected holder to keep hot foods hot.

- Stay hydrated. Fluids, for example, water, unsweetened tea, coffee, 100% natural product juice, just as hydrating foods, for example, leafy foods help keep our joints, organs, and cerebrum working appropriately. Before snatching a fatty treat, drink a glass of water. In many cases, we believe we're eager, yet we're dried out. That glass of water may spare you additional calories you honestly would prefer not to devour.

- Did you realize that rest is an essential part of a sound way of life – and even our midriff size? There's a relationship between the measure of rest we get with our weight file. On the off chance that you find you're not getting 7-8 hours rest for every night, do a daily practice before sleep time and set up for a decent night's rest. Start by turning off the TV, PC, and wireless, ensure your room is dull and relaxed, and afterward close your eyes and make the most of your merited magnificence rest.

Perfect Weight Loss Strategies:

Get any diet book, and it will profess to hold every one of the responses to effectively losing all the weight you need—and keeping it off. Some case the key is to eat less and practice more, others that low fat is the best way to go, while others endorse removing carbs. All in all, what would be a good idea for you to accept? The truth of the situation here is that there is no "one size fits all" solution for longlasting weight loss regime. What works for one individual may not work for you, since our bodies react distinctively to various foods, contingent upon hereditary qualities and other wellbeing factors. To discover the technique for weight reduction that is directly for you will probably require some investment and require tolerance, duty, and some experimentation with various foods and diets.

While a few people react well to checking calories or comparable prohibitive strategies, others respond better to having more opportunity in planning their health improvement plans. Being allowed to just stay away from seared foods or cut back on refined carbs can set them up for progress. Along these lines, don't get excessively debilitated if a diet that worked for another person doesn't work for you. What's more, don't pummel yourself if a diet demonstrates unreasonably prohibitive for you to stay with. Eventually, a diet is directly for you if it's one you can remain with after some time.

Keep in mind: while there's no simple fix to getting thinner, there are a lot of steps you can take to build up a more beneficial association with food, control enthusiastic triggers to gorging, and accomplish a solid weight.

These procedures have been demonstrated to work consummately for weight reduction:

- Understand Some Calories:

A few specialists accept that effectively dealing with your weight boils down to a straightforward condition: If you eat fewer calories than you consume, you shed pounds. Sounds simple, isn't that so? At that point for what reason is shedding pounds so hard?

- Weight misfortune is certainly not a straight occasion after some time. When you cut calories, you may drop weight for an initial couple of weeks, for instance, and afterward, something changes. You eat a similar number of calories; however, you lose less weight or no weight by any means. That is because when you shed pounds, you're losing water and lean tissue just as fat, your digestion eases back, and your body changes in different ways. In this way, to keep dropping weight every week, you have to continue cutting calories.

- A calorie isn't constantly a calorie. Consuming a hundred calories of high fructose contained in corn syrup, for instance, can variably have an effect on your body than consuming a hundred calories of broccoli. The stunt for continued weight reduction is to discard the foods that are stuffed with calories yet don't make you feel full (like sweets) and supplant them with food sources that top you off without being stacked with calories (like vegetables).

- Many people don't necessarily eat just to quench hunger. They likewise go to food for solace or to alleviate pressure —which can rapidly wreck any weight-reduction plan.

Watch Your Carb Intake:

An alternate method for survey weight reduction distinguishes the issue as not one of expending an excessive number of calories, but instead how the body aggregates fat in the wake of devouring sugars—precisely the job of the hormone insulin. When you eat supper, sugars from the food enter your bloodstream as glucose. To hold your blood sugar levels in line, your body consistently consumes off this glucose before it consumes off fat from a dinner.

If you eat a sugar-rich feast (heaps of pasta, rice, bread, or French fries, for instance), your body discharges insulin to help with the inundation of this glucose into your blood. Just as directing blood sugar levels, insulin completes two things: It keeps your fat cells from discharging fat for the body to copy as fuel (since its need is to copy off the glucose) and it makes increasingly fat cells for putting away everything that your body can't copy off. The outcome is that you put on weight and your body presently requires more fuel to consume, so you eat more. Since insulin consumes starches, you need carbs, thus starts an endless loop of devouring carbs and putting on weight. To get in shape, the thinking goes, you have to break this cycle by diminishing carbs.

Most low-carb diets supporter supplanting carbs with protein and fat, which could have some negative long-haul impacts on

117

your wellbeing. If you do attempt a low-carb diet, you can diminish your dangers and point of confinement your admission of immersed and trans fats by picking lean meats, fish and veggie lover wellsprings of protein, low-fat dairy items, and eating a lot of verdant green and non-bland vegetables.

- Watch Your Fat Intake:

It's a pillar of numerous diets: on the off chance that you would prefer not to get fat, don't eat fat. Stroll down any supermarket passageway, and you'll be assaulted with decreased fatty tidbits, dairy, and bundled suppers. In any case, while our low-fat alternatives have detonated, so have weight rates. All in all, for what reason haven't low-fat diets worked for a higher amount of people?

- Not all fat is awful. Sound or high fats can control your weight, as deal with your states of mind and battle fatigue. Unsaturated fats found in avocados, nuts, seeds, soy milk, tofu, and fatty fish can help top you off, while including a little tasty olive oil to a plate of vegetables, for instance, can make it simpler to eat well food and improve the general nature of your diet.

- We regularly make an inappropriate exchange off. A large number of us tragically swap fat for the vacant calories of sugar and refined starches. Rather than eating whole-fat yogurt, for instance, we eat low-or no-fat forms that are pressed with sugar to compensate for the loss of taste. Or on the other hand, we swap our fatty breakfast bacon for a biscuit or doughnut that causes fast spikes in blood sugar.

- Be Consistent in Keeping the Weight Off:

You may have heard the broadly cited measurement that 95% of individuals who get more fit on a diet will recover it inside a couple of years—or even months. While there isn't much hard proof to help that guarantee, the facts confirm that many weight reduction plans bomb in the long haul. Frequently that is just because diets that are too prohibitive are challenging to keep up after some time. In any case, that doesn't mean your weight reduction endeavors are destined to disappointment — a long way from it.

Since it was built up in 1994, The National Weight Control Registry (NWCR) in the United States, has followed more than 10,000 people who have lost noteworthy measures of weight and kept it off for extensive periods. The investigation has discovered that members who've been fruitful in keeping up their weight reduction share some regular procedures. Whatever diet you use to get in shape in any case, receiving these propensities may assist you with keeping it off:

- Stay physically dynamic. Effective dieters in the NWCR study practice for around an hour, commonly strolling.

- Keep a food log. Recording what you eat each day keeps you responsible and spurred.

- Eat breakfast each day. Most ordinarily in the investigation, it's grain and organic product. Having breakfast supports digestion and fights off craving later in the day.

- Eat more fiber and less unfortunate fat than the run of the American mill diet.

- Regularly check the scale. Gauging yourself week by week may assist you with detecting any little puts on in weight, empowering you to make a remedial move before the issue heightens expeditiously.

- Watch less TV. Reducing the time spent sitting before a screen can be a crucial piece of receiving an increasingly dynamic way of life and counteracting weight gain.

Quick Recipes for the Mediterranean Diet

The Mediterranean diet has consistently positioned most noteworthy among prominent foods — and all things considered. It's one of the most adaptable, flavorful menus around, urging you to load up your plate with beautiful produce, heart-solid fish, and entire grains. Here are 40 Mediterranean diet plans that will set you up for feel-great eating. These are breakfast, lunch, supper, and pastry fast plans that will set you up for the diet as quickly as time permits.

Breakfast:

• Mediterranean Scrambled Eggs:
Fried eggs are the simplest things to make, and this heart-solid breaky packs in a full serving of veggies like yellow pepper, cherry tomatoes, spring onion, and dark olives (well, in fact, a natural product!). Toss the blend onto a bit of whole-grain toast, and you'll be as brilliant as the Mediterranean sun.

Per serving: 249 calories, 17 g fat (4 g soaked), 13 g carbs, 4 g sugar, 334 mg sodium, 3 g fiber, 14 g protein. Planning Time: 5 mins. Cook Time: 10 mins.

Ingredients: 1 tbsp oil; 1 yellow pepper, diced; 2 spring onions, cut; 8 cherry tomatoes, quartered; 2 tbsp cut dark olives; 1 tbsp tricks; 4 eggs; 1/4 tsp dried oregano; Black pepper; Fresh parsley, to serve (discretionary)

Directions:

121

- Heat the oil in a skillet, and include the diced pepper and slashed spring onions. Cook for a couple of minutes over medium warmth, until somewhat delicate. Include the quartered tomatoes, olives and tricks, and cook for one increasingly minute.

- Crack the eggs into the dish, and quickly scramble with a spoon or spatula. Include the oregano and a lot of dark pepper, and continue mixing until the eggs are thoroughly cooked. Serve warm, bested with fresh parsley whenever wanted.

- Watermelon, Feta, and Balsamic Pizza

You'll score all the Instagram likes with this morning meal pizza that blends the reciprocal kinds of feta, mint, olives, and balsamic. Get a couple reviving cuts before your regularly scheduled drive.

Per serving: 90 calories, 3 g fat (1 g immersed), 14 g carbs, 12 g sugar, 148 mg sodium, 1 g fiber, 2 g protein.

Ingredients: 1 watermelon cut, cut 1-inch thick from the focal point of the amplest section; 1 oz disintegrated Feta cheddar; 5 to 6 Kalamata Olives, chopped; 1 tsp mint leaves; 1/2 tbsp balsamic coating

Directions:
- Slice the most extensive piece of a round watermelon down the middle. Lay the level side down on a cutting board and cut a 1-inch thick cut from every half. Cut every half into four wedges.

- Place them on a round dish like a pizza and top with cheddar, olives, balsamic coating, and mint leaves.

- Low Carb Egg Muffins Topped with Special Ham

It turns out you can, in any case, get your biscuit fix while sticking to a sound, high-protein diet. This one has every one of the makings of a satisfying breakfast, and it doesn't hurt that they're beautiful to take a gander at, as well.

Per serving: 109 calories, 6 g fat (2 g soaked), 2 g carbs, 1 g sugar, 423 mg sodium, 2 g fiber, 9 g protein

Ingredients:

9 Slices of slim-cut store ham; 1/2 Cup Canned cooked red pepper, cut + extra for embellishment; 1/3 Cup Fresh spinach, minced; 1/4 Cup Feta cheddar, disintegrated; 5 Large eggs; Pinch of salt; Pinch of pepper; 1/2 Tbsps Pesto sauce; Fresh basil for trimming

Directions:

- Preheat your stove to 400 degrees. Liberally shower a biscuit tin with cooking splash.

- Line every biscuit tin with 1.5 bits of ham, ensuring you don't leave gaps for the egg blend to burst out of.

- Place a tad of cooked red pepper in the base of every biscuit tin.

- Place 1 Tbsp of minced spinach over every red pepper.

- Top the pepper and spinach off with a loading 1/2 Tbsp of disintegrated feta cheddar.

- In a medium bowl, whisk together the eggs salt and pepper. Partition the egg blend equitably among the six biscuit tins.

- Bake for 15-17 minutes until the eggs are puffy and feel set.

- Remove each cup from the biscuit tin and top with 1/4 tsp pesto sauce, extra simmered red pepper cuts, and new basil.

- Avocado Tomato Gouda Socca Pizza:

Avocado toast is necessarily required on this diet; however, this formula takes it up an indent with sans gluten chickpea flour as its base, in addition to grew grains and gouda to balance the flavors and nourishing profile.

Per serving: 416 calories, 25 g fat (5 g immersed), 37 g carbs, 7 g sugar, 257 mg sodium, 10 g fiber, 15 g protein.

Ingredients:
- For the Socca Pizza Crust:

1/4 cup chickpea/garbanzo bean flour; 1/4 cup cold water; 1/4 tsp ocean salt and pepper each (to taste); 2 tbsp olive or avocado oil (1 tbsp for warming skillet); 1 tsp minced; Garlic (2 cloves); 1 tsp of Onion powder or some other herbed flavoring of decision; 10 to 12 inch Pan to warm in stove (cast iron works extraordinarily.)

- Socca Pizza Toppings:

1 Roma tomato cut; 1/2 avocado; 2 oz Gouda (cut dainty); 1/4 to 1/3 cup Tomato sauce; 2–3 tbsp cleaved green onion/scallion; Sprouted greens (onion greens, kale, or broccoli) to top; Extra Salt/pepper to sprinkle on top; Red pepper drops.

Guidance:

- First Mix your flour, 2 tbsp olive oil, water, and herbs/flavoring together. Rush until smooth. It's ideal for giving it a chance to sit for 15-20 minutes at room temperature.

- While the player is sitting, preheat broiler to cook. Spot your container on the stove to warm for 10 minutes.

- While the dish is preheating, slash/cut your vegetables. Put in a safe spot.

- Using stove gloves, evacuate dish following 10 minutes.

- Add 1 tbsp of oil to the dish and whirl it around to cover the container

- Gently pour in your chickpea/socca hitter. Tilt skillet, so the hitter fills and is even.

- Turn stove down to 425F and spot skillet back in the grill for 5-8 minutes or somewhere in the vicinity just until the hitter is set. On the off chance that you are utilizing an enormous container, the pizza will be more slender and will most likely prepare quicker, so check at 5 minutes.

- Remove from grill.

- Spread the tomato sauce on top. At that point include your cut tomato and avocado. Spot your gouda cuts over the

125

tomato and avocado. Green onion can go on the top, or you can stand by to include crisp last.

- Place back in a grill for 10-15 minutes until cheddar is softened and the socca bread is firm and darker on the outside.

- Remove from the grill. You ought to have the option to slide the pizza covering onto a stone or warmth safe surface.

- Add a lot of sprouts/microgreens on top than any extra fixings. Like more onion, salt/pepper to taste, and red pepper drops.

- Drizzle olive oil on top. Cut and serve.

- Gingerbread Breakfast Quinoa Bake with Banana

This heart-sound breakfast incorporates entire grains, natural product, and a lot of protein-pressed nuts—all marks of a Mediterranean breakfast. It possesses a flavor like absolutely debauched solace nourishment that can likewise fulfill your craving for a noontime treat.

Per serving: 213 calories, 4 g fat (0 g immersed), 41 g carbs, 18 g sugar, 211 mg sodium, 4 g fiber, 5 g protein.

Ingredients: 3 cups Medium over-ready ONE Bananas pounded (just shy of 1/2 or 370g); 1/4 Cup Molasses; 1/4 Cup Pure maple syrup; 1 Tbsp Cinnamon

2 tsp Raw vanilla concentrate; 1 tsp Ground ginger; 1 tsp Ground cloves; 1/2 tsp Ground allspice; 1/2 tsp Salt; 1 Cup Quinoa

uncooked; 2 1/2 Cups Unsweetened vanilla almond milk; 1/4 Cup Slivered almonds.

Guidelines:

- In the base of a 2 1/2-3 quart goulash dish, blend the squashed banana, molasses, maple syrup, cinnamon, vanilla concentrate, ginger, cloves, allspice, and salt until all around blended. Include the quinoa and mix until the quinoa is uniformly conveyed in the banana blend.

- Whisk in the almond milk until all around consolidated. Spread and refrigerate medium-term.

- In the morning, heat your stove to 350 degrees and whisk the quinoa blend to ensure it hasn't settled to the base.

- Cover the dish with tinfoil and prepare until the fluid is ingested, and the highest point of the quinoa is set, around 60 minutes - to 1 hour and 15 mins.

- Turn your stove to high sear, reveal the container, sprinkle with sliced almonds, and daintily press them into the quinoa. Cook until the almonds turn brilliant dark-colored, around 2-4 minutes. Watch intently as they consume rapidly!

- Let cool for 10 minutes at that point, serve and eat.

- Greek Goddess Bowl

Veggie lover tzatziki and red pepper hemp tabbouleh top fresh prepared chickpeas for a fantastic mash in this exquisite breakfast.

127

Per serving: 519 calories, 35 g fat (20 g soaked), 50 g carbs, 20 g sugar, 609 mg sodium, 13 g fiber, 12 g protein.

Ingredients:
- CHICKPEAS:

1 15-ounce can chickpeas (washed, depleted and dried well on a towel); 1 Tbsp oil (coconut or avocado are best/discard if dodging oil); 1 Tbsp Shawarma Spice Blend (or comparative flavors you have close by); 1 Tbsp maple syrup or coconut sugar (if maintaining a strategic distance from sugar, overlook); 1/4 tsp ocean salt

- BOWL:

3/4 cup Vegan Tzatziki; 1 clump Red Pepper Hemp Tabbouleh (or sub hacked parsley); 1/2 cup green or kalamata olives (set and split/cleaved); 1/2 cup cherry tomatoes (divided); 1 medium cucumber (meagerly cut); 1 medium carrot (discretionary/cut daintily on a corner to corner into "chips").

Guidelines:
- Preheat grill to 375 degrees F (190 C) and set out a preparing sheet.

- Add washed, dried chickpeas to a blending bowl alongside oil, Shawarma Spice Blend, maple syrup, and salt. Hurl to consolidate.

- Add prepared chickpeas to the heating sheet. Prepare for 20-23 minutes or until the chickpeas are somewhat firm and brilliant darker. Expel from broiler and put in a safe spot.

- Assemble bowl by partitioning tzatziki, tabbouleh (or parsley), olives, tomatoes, cucumber, and carrots (discretionary) between two serving bowls. Top with cooked chickpeas and trimming with new lemon juice.

- This bowl is heavenly as may be; it would likewise match well with my 4-fixing Garlic Dill Sauce or my Tahini Dressing!

- Best when crisp, yet you can store scraps (independently) up to 3-4 days in the fridge. Store remaining chickpeas individually in a fixed holder at room temperature as long as three days or in the cooler as long as a multi-month.

- Greek Guacamole

Avocado toast is almost an ideal nourishment all alone, yet this formula enables you to top your morning (entire grain!) toast with that additional Mediterranean edge. In case you're into sun-dried tomatoes, kalamata olives, and crisp hacked parsley, you'll need this plunge to be the main thing you eat each morning.

Per serving: 110 calories, 10 g fat (2 g soaked), 6 g carbs, 1 g sugar, 54 mg sodium, 4 g fiber, 1 g protein.

Ingredients:
2 huge ready avocados (split, pit evacuated); 2 Tbsp lemon juice; 1 storing Tbsp hacked sun-dried tomatoes; 3 Tbsp diced available cherry tomato; 1/4 cup diced red onion; 1 tsp dried oregano (or sub new); 2 Tbsp crisp cleaved parsley; 4 entire kalamata olives (hollowed and slashed/discretionary); 1 squeeze every ocean salt and dark pepper.

Guidelines:

- Add avocado and lemon juice to an enormous blending bowl and utilize a potato masher, baked good shaper, or huge fork to squash and blend.

- Add residual fixings (olives are discretionary), and blend to consolidate (see photograph). Test and include salt and pepper if necessary.

- Adjust different flavors if necessary, including more lemon for acidity, sun-dried tomato for more profound tomato enhance, onion for crunch/zest, or parsley or oregano.

- Enjoy promptly with pita, pita chips, or vegetables! Best when crisp, however, remains to keep in the fridge for 2-3 days.

- Feta Frozen Yogurt

Feta and Greek yogurt are the ideal methods to get your calcium and protein, while a portion of nectar gives natural sweetness and follow minerals.

Per serving: 161 calories, 10 g fat (7 g immersed), 7 g carbs, 12 g sugar, 329 mg sodium, 0 g fiber, 7 g protein.

Ingredients:
One cup plain Greek yogurt 200 g; 1/2 cup feta cheddar 50 g; 1 Tbsp nectar 15 ml.

Guidelines:

- Freeze: In a nourishment processor or blender, join all fixings until smooth. Fill a deep dish (it shouldn't be an extremely thick layer) and stop until strong.

- Blend: Break solidified mixture into pieces and include once again into your blender, alongside a couple of tablespoons of water or milk. Barrage until smooth and creamy, scratching down the sides as expected to get everything mixed. Serve sprinkled with nectar.

- Greek Omelet Casserole

Prepare a significant cluster toward the beginning of the day and re-heat it the following day (either for breakfast or supper!). With flavors like sundried tomato-mixed feta cheddar and new dill, you can't turn out badly with this dish, regardless of the hour of the day.

Per serving: 196 calories, 12 g fat (4 g immersed), 5 g carbs, 3 g sugar, 536 mg sodium, 1 g fiber, 10 g protein.

Ingredients:
12 enormous eggs; 2 cups entire milk; 8 ounces crisp spinach; 2 cloves garlic, minced; 12 ounces artichoke serving of mixed greens (with olives and peppers) depleted and hacked; 5 ounces sun-dried tomato feta cheddar, disintegrated; 1 tablespoon new slashed dill (1 teaspoon dried dill); 1 teaspoon dried oregano; 1 teaspoon lemon pepper; 1 teaspoon salt; 4 teaspoons olive oil, isolated.

Guidelines:
131

- Preheat grill to 375 degrees F. Slash the fresh herbs and artichoke plate of mixed greens.

- Set a skillet over medium warmth and include one tablespoon olive oil. Sauté the spinach and garlic until withered, around 3 minutes.

- Oil a 9x13 inch heating dish and layer the spinach and artichoke serving of mixed greens equally in the bowl.

- In a medium bowl, whisk together the eggs, milk, herbs, salt and lemon pepper.

- Pour the egg blend over vegetables and sprinkle with feta cheddar. Heat in the focal point of the broiler for 35-40 minutes until firm in the middle.

- Cauliflower Fritters with Hummus

Oxygen is essential to the human being because it is what keeps us living. That also can be said about hummus in the Mediterranean diet. The veggie existing apart from everything else (taking a gander at you, cauliflower) gets a beautiful overhaul plunged in chickpea goodness. What's more, it's necessarily the simplest method to begin your vacation day on the correct plant-based note.

Per serving: 333 calories, 13 g fat (2 g immersed), 45 g carbs, 9 g sugar, 323 mg sodium, 13 g fiber, 14 g protein.

Ingredients:
2 15-ounce jars chickpeas, partitioned; 2 1/2 tablespoons olive oil, isolated, in addition to additional for broiling; 1 cup onion,

cleaved, around 1/2 a little onion; 2 tablespoons garlic, minced; 2 cups cauliflower, cut into small pieces, approximately 1/2 a considerable head; 1/2 teaspoon salt; dark pepper; hummus, ff decision, for fixing; diced green onion, for enhancement.

Guidance:

- Preheat your broiler to 400°F.

- Rinse and channel one jar of the chickpeas and spot them on a paper towel, getting them dry thoroughly. Spot the chickpeas into a considerable bowl, expelling any of the free skins that fall off, and hurl with one tablespoon of olive oil. Spread them onto a large skillet, being mindful so as not to pack them, and sprinkle with salt and pepper.

- Bake the chickpeas for 20 minutes, mix, and afterward prepare an extra 5-10 minutes until fresh.

- Once the chickpeas are broiled, move them into a massive food processor and procedure until separated and brittle. Try not to transform them into flour, as you need to leave some surface. Spot into a little bowl and put in a safe spot.

- Heat the staying 1/2 tablespoon of olive oil in a large dish on medium-high heat. Include the onion and garlic and cook until gently brilliant darker, around 2 minutes. Include the cleaved cauliflower and cook an extra 2 minutes, until the cauliflower is likewise bright.

- Turn the warmth down to low and cover the skillet. Cook until the cauliflower is fork delicate and the onions are brilliant dark-colored and caramelized, mixing now and then. This takes around 3-5 minutes.

133

- Transfer the cauliflower blend into the nourishment processor. Channel and flush the remaining container of chickpeas and include it into the nourishment processor, alongside the salt and a decent squeeze of pepper. Mix until smooth, and the blend begins to transform into a ball, halting to scratch down the sides as vital.

- Transfer the cauliflower blend into an enormous bowl and include 1/2 cup of the cooked chickpea scraps (you don't utilize the majority of the morsels; however, it's simpler to separate them when you have a more significant sum.) Stir until very much joined.

- Pour merely enough oil to gently cover the base of a large container and warmth on medium warmth. Cook the patties until brilliant darker, around 2-3 minutes, flip and cook once more. It's simplest to cook a couple at once and work in different groups.

- Top with hummus, green onion and eat.

Plans for Lunch:

- Greek Chicken and Rice Skillet

Ingredients:

6 chicken thighs; Kosher salt and crisply ground dark pepper; 1 teaspoon dried oregano; 1 teaspoon garlic powder; 3 lemons; 2 tablespoons extra-virgin olive oil; ½ red onion, minced; 2 garlic cloves, minced; 1 cup long-grain rice; 2½ cups chicken soup; 1 tablespoon hacked new oregano, in addition to additional for decorating; 1 cup green olives; ½ cup disintegrated feta cheddar; ⅓ cup fresh cleaved new parsley.

Directions:

- Preheat the stove to 375°F. Season the chicken thighs with salt and pepper. In a little bowl, mix the dried oregano, garlic powder and the get-up-and-go of 1 lemon. Rub the blend equitably over the chicken.

- Heat the olive oil in a large stove safe skillet over medium warmth. Include the chicken, skin side down, and sear until the chicken is very much cooked 7 to 9 minutes. Evacuate to a plate and save.

- Add the onion and garlic to the skillet and sauté until translucent, around 5 minutes. Blend in the rice and sauté for one moment; season with salt.

- Add the chicken soup and carry the blend to a stew. Blend in the new oregano and the juice of the zested lemon. Cut the staying two lemons and put in a safe spot.

- Nestle the chicken, skin side up, into the rice blend. Move the skillet to the grill and cook until the rice has consumed the majority of the fluid, and the chicken is thoroughly cooked 20 to 25 minutes.

- Turn on the grill and orchestrate the lemon cuts over the chicken. Cook the skillet until the lemons are softly singed and the chicken skin is fresh around 3 minutes.

- Add the olives and feta to the skillet, decorate with fresh parsley, and serve right away.

- Heirloom Tomato and Cucumber Toast

Ingredients:

One little legacy tomato, diced; 1 Persian cucumber, diced; 1 teaspoon extra-virgin olive oil; Pinch of dried oregano; Kosher salt and newly ground dark pepper; 2 teaspoons low-fat whipped cream cheddar; 2 pieces Trader Joe's Whole Grain Crispbread; 1 teaspoon balsamic coating

Guidelines:

- In a medium bowl, join the tomato, cucumber, olive oil, and oregano; season with salt and pepper.

- Smear the cream cheddar on the bread and top with the tomato-cucumber blend and the balsamic coating.

- Mini Chicken Shawarma

Ingredients:

CHICKEN: 1-pound chicken strips; ¼ cup extra-virgin olive oil; Zest and squeeze of 1 lemon; 2 teaspoons garlic powder; 1 teaspoon ground cumin; ¾ teaspoon ground coriander; ½ teaspoon smoked paprika; 1 teaspoon crisply ground dark pepper

SAUCE: 1¼ cups Greek yogurt; 1 tablespoon lemon juice; 1 garlic clove, ground; ¼ cup cleaved crisp parsley; 2 tablespoons hacked new dill; Kosher salt and newly ground dark pepper; ½ red onion, meagerly cut; 4 leaves romaine lettuce, destroyed; ½ English cucumber, daintily sliced; 2 tomatoes, slashed; 16 smaller than usual pita bread.

Directions:

- MAKE THE CHICKEN: Place the chicken in a substantial resealable plastic sack. In a little bowl, whisk together the olive oil, lemon pizzazz, lemon juice, garlic powder, cumin, coriander, paprika and pepper to join. Empty the marinade into the pack, seal and hurl the chicken well to cover. Give the chicken a chance to marinate for 30 minutes to 60 minutes.

- MAKE THE SAUCE: While the chicken marinates, blend the Greek yogurt, lemon juice and garlic in a medium bowl. Mix in the parsley and dill; season with salt and pepper. Spread and refrigerate.

- Heat a large skillet over medium warmth. Expel the chicken from the marinade, giving the overabundance trickle a chance to off, and cook until it's very much seared on the two sides and thoroughly cooked, around 4 minutes for each team. Slash it into scaled-down strips.

- To gather, separate the chicken, onion, lettuce, cucumber, and tomato uniformly among the pitas.

- Mezze Plate with Toasted Za'atar Pita Bread

Ingredients:

Four entire wheat pita rounds; 4 tablespoons extra-virgin olive oil; 4 teaspoons za'atar; 1 cup Greek yogurt; Kosher salt and naturally ground dark pepper; 1 cup hummus; 1 cup marinated artichoke hearts; 1 cup cut cooked red peppers; 2 cups grouped olives; 2 cups cherry tomatoes; 4 ounces salami.

Guidance:

- Heat a large skillet over medium-high heat. Brush the two sides of every pita with olive oil and season with the za'atar.

- Working in bunches, add the pita to the skillet and toast until brilliant dark-colored, around 2 minutes for every side. Cut every pita into quarters.

- Season the Greek yogurt with salt and pepper.

- To gather, partition the pitas, Greek yogurt, hummus, artichoke hearts, cooked red peppers, olives, tomatoes and salami among four plates.

- Cold Lemon Zoodles

Ingredients:

One lemon, zested and squeezed; ½ teaspoon Dijon mustard; ½ teaspoon garlic powder; ⅓ cup olive oil; Salt and newly ground dark pepper; 3 medium zucchini, cut into noodles; 1 bundle radishes, meagerly cut; 1 tablespoon hacked new thyme.

Guidance:

- In a little bowl, whisk the lemon get-up-and-go, lemon juice, mustard and garlic powder to join.

- Gradually include the olive oil and speed to consolidate. Season with salt and pepper.

- In a large bowl, hurl the zucchini noodles with the radishes. Include the dressing and throw until the veggies are all around covered.

- Serve promptly, embellished with new thyme.

- Harissa Potato Salad

Ingredients:

1/2 lbs child potatoes (leave the skins on); 2 tablespoons harissa glue; 6 ounces low-fat or non-fat Greek yogurt; 1/4 tsp. Salt; 1/4 tsp. Pepper; Juice of 1 lemon; 1/4 cup finely diced red onion; 1/4 cup new cilantro or parsley, generally hacked.

Guidance:

- Place the potatoes in a huge pot and spread them with 1-to 2-creeps of chilly, salted water. Heat the water to the point of boiling over medium-high heat. At that point cook the potatoes, revealed, until they are fork delicate, around 9-11 minutes. Channel the potatoes and put them aside to cool somewhat.

- Meanwhile, in a little bowl whisk together the harissa, Greek yogurt, salt, pepper, and lemon juice.

- Transfer the still-warm potatoes to a huge bowl. Include the dressing and crease it in tenderly until the vegetables are very much covered. At that point cautiously overlap in the diced red onion and herbs.

- Serve promptly while still warm, at room temperature or in the wake of being chilled.

- Leftovers can be put away in an impenetrable holder in your cooler for 2-3 days.

- Greek Fattoush Salad:

139

Ingredients:

For the plate of mixed greens: 2 entire wheat pitas or flatbread rounds (white works fine as well); 2 tablespoons olive oil; 1/4 teaspoon genuine salt; 4 cups cleaved romaine lettuce; 1 medium cucumber, stripped, quartered, and cut; 1 yellow ringer pepper, cut into 3/4-inch lumps; 1/2 16 ounces (1 cup) cherry tomatoes, divided; 1/2 little red onion, daintily cut; 1/2 cup level Italian parsley leaves; 1/2 cup Kalamata olives, split; 3/4 cup disintegrated feta cheddar.

For the dressing: 1/3 cup olive oil; 2 tablespoons red wine vinegar; 1 little clove garlic, minced; 1/2 teaspoon dried oregano; 1/4 teaspoon suitable salt; 1/8 teaspoon naturally ground dark pepper.

Guidelines:
- Preheat grill to 350°F.

- Cut the pitas fifty-fifty and spot them on a heating sheet. Prepare, turning once, until brilliant dark colored and toasted, 10-15 minutes. Let cool. Break or cut the toasted pitas into reduced down (1-inch) pieces. Add them to a medium bowl and sprinkle two tablespoons of olive oil over the bread. Hurl to cover. Sprinkle with suitable salt and hurl again to appropriate. Put in a safe spot.

- To an enormous bowl, including the lettuce, cucumber, ringer pepper, tomatoes, onion, parsley, and olives. Hurl.

- Make the vinaigrette. To a little bowl, including the 1/3 cup olive oil, vinegar, garlic, oregano, salt, and pepper. Race until mixed.

- Add the pita bread pieces and the feta to the serving of mixed greens. Sprinkle the vinaigrette over the top. Hurl delicately to join. Serve right away.

- Greek Lemon Chicken Soup

Ingredients:

2 tablespoons olive oil, isolated; 1-pound boneless, skinless chicken thighs, cut into 1-inch pieces; Kosher salt and newly ground dark pepper; 4 cloves garlic, minced; 1 onion, diced; 3 carrots, stripped and diced; 2 stalks celery, diced; 1/2 teaspoon dried thyme; 8 cups chicken stock; 2 straight leaves; 2 (15.5 ounce) jars cannellini beans, flushed and depleted; 4 cups infant spinach; 2 tablespoons newly pressed lemon juice, or more, to taste; 2 tablespoons slashed crisp parsley leaves; 2 tablespoons hacked new dill.

Guidelines:

- Heat 1 tablespoon olive oil in an enormous stockpot or Dutch grill over medium warmth. For a good taste, give the chicken thighs a good seasoning with pepper and salt. Add chicken to the stockpot and cook until brilliant, around 2-3 minutes; put in a safe spot.

- Add staying one tablespoon oil to the stockpot. Include garlic, onion, carrots, and celery. Cook, blending incidentally, until delicate, around 3-4 minutes. Blend in thyme until fragrant, around one moment.

- Whisk in chicken stock and straight leaves. Heat to the point of boiling; decrease warmth and mix in cannellini beans and chicken, mixing incidentally, until marginally thickened, around 10-15 minutes.

- Stir in spinach until withered, around 2 minutes. Mix in lemon juice, parsley, and dill; season with salt and pepper, to taste.

- Serve right away.

- Mediterranean Chicken Tacos

Ingredients:

8 delicate taco shells; 2-3 chicken bosoms defrosted and cut into scaled-down pieces; 1/2 cup grape tomatoes cut; 1/4 cup red onion cut; 2/3 cup feta cheddar; 1 cup hummus locally acquired or this formula less the sesame seeds; Tzatziki sauce;; 6 garlic cloves; 1/2 cup cucumber; Juice from 1/2 lemon; 2 tsp new dill; 2 mint leaves; half cup of plain Greek yogurt; Enough salt and pepper to enhance taste.

Guidance:
- Heat a large skillet with 1-2 tbsp of oil and after that cook chicken in skillet until it's finished.

- While chicken is cooking, make the tzatziki sauce and the hummus. For the tzatziki sauce: consolidate garlic, cucumber, lemon, dill, and mint in a blender and heartbeat for 5-10 seconds. Fill an enormous bowl and mix in yogurt by hand until everything is joined; saved.

- Also, make sure to leave up the tomatoes and onion while the chicken is cooking.

- Once the chicken is done, empty it into the bowl of tzatziki sauce and mix until chicken is well-covered.

- Heat taco shells in a skillet until warm and afterward fill them with hummus, chicken, and vegetables.

- Warm Potato Salad with Smoked Mackerel Recipe

Ingredients:
300g (10oz) new potatoes, split or cut into thick cuts; About 150g (5oz) broccoli, cut into smallish florets; 2 teaspoons juice vinegar or wine vinegar; 1-2 teaspoons coarse-grain mustard; 4-6 teaspoons olive oil; 3-4 cooked infant beetroot, quartered

Two smoked mackerel fillets, complete load about 150g (5oz)

Directions:
- Add the potatoes to a dish of bubbling water and cook for 10 minutes, at that point include the broccoli florets and cook for 2-3 minutes.

- Whisk the vinegar and mustard with the oil to make a dressing.

- Drain the vegetables well, tip into a bowl, and blend in the dressing to cover well.

- Add the beetroot quarters and chipped mackerel.

Plans for Dinner

- Easy One-Pan Mediterranean Cod

Ingredients:

2 tbsp olive oil; 1 little onion cut; 2 cups cut fennel; 3 huge cloves garlic cleaved; 1 14.5 ounces can diced tomato; 1 cup diced crisp tomatoes; 2 cups destroyed kale; 1/2 cup water; squeeze of squashed red pepper; 2 tsp new oregano or 1/2 tsp dried oregano; 1 cup oil relieved dark olives; 1 lb. cod cut into four parts; 1/8 tsp salt; 1/4 tsp dark pepper; 1/4 tsp fennel seeds discretionary; 1 tsp orange pizzazz; crisp oregano fennel fronds, orange get-up-and-go, olive oil.

Directions:

- In a considerable skillet (in a perfect world with high sides) over medium warmth, cook onion, fennel, and garlic in olive oil for 8 minutes, season with salt and pepper (around 1/4 tsp of each). Include canned diced tomato, crisp tomato, kale, and water. Blend well and cook for 12 minutes. Include squashed red pepper, fresh oregano, and olives.

- Prepare fish, season with salt, pepper, orange get-up-and-go, and fennel seeds (discretionary). Settle fish into kale tomato stewing blend. Spread skillet and cook for 10 minutes.

- Remove from warmth, and finish with fennel fronds, all the newer oregano, increasingly orange pizzazz, and a sprinkle of olive oil on top.

- Serve right away.

- Smooth meatball formula with Bucatini pasta formula

Ingredients:

400g unfenced pork and apple frankfurters; 2tbsp olive oil; 1 little onion, hacked; 1 garlic clove, squashed; ½ a new or dried bean stew, finely slashed bunch of enormous basil leaves; 1 x 400g tinned plummed tomatoes; 2tbsp tomato puree; 1tbsp dried oregano; 1tbsp balsamic vinegar; 300g Bucatini pasta; 40g ground Parmesan cheddar, to serve.

Directions:

- Squeeze the meat from the hotdogs into a bowl and include 1tbsp of the slashed onion. Season well and join ultimately. With clammy hands structure the blend into 12 equivalent estimated meatballs. Refrigerate for 20-30 minutes – this will enable them to solidify.

- Meanwhile, put the oil in a skillet on a medium-high heat. Cook the rest of the onion for 5-7 minutes, until delicate and softly brilliant. Include the garlic and stew, and when they are shaded include the large basil leaves.

- Tip in the tomatoes, puree, dried oregano, and balsamic vinegar. Bring to a stew and cook for an additional couple of minutes.

- Fry the meatballs on medium-high heat until hued and cooked through. When cooked, add the meatballs to the tomato sauce. Cook the pasta in bubbling salted water as indicated by bundle guidelines, at that point channel and return the pasta to the skillet. Include a large portion of the pasta sauce and blend. Partition the pasta among plates and spoon the meatballs and remaining sauce on top with a liberal grinding or Parmesan.

- Chicken and tomato pasta heat formula

145

Ingredients:

2tbsp olive oil; 1 onion, stripped and finely hacked; 2 garlic cloves, stripped and squashed; 400g skinless chicken bosom filet, cut into pieces; 400g can slash tomatoes; 2tbsp sun-dried tomato glue; Pinch of sugar; 2tbsp cleaved crisp basil, in addition to leaves to embellish; Salt and newly ground dark pepper; 400g dried pasta shapes; 150g prepared ground mozzarella cheddar.

Directions:

- Heat the oil in a large skillet and fry the onion and garlic for 5 mins until mollified. Include the chicken and fry for a further 5 mins, until carmelized everywhere. Blend in the cleaved tomatoes, tomato glue, sugar, and basil. Season with salt and naturally ground dark pepper and stew delicately for 15 mins.

- Meanwhile, heat the pasta shapes in a large dish of gently salted water as indicated by the bundle guidelines. Preheat the grill to 220°C/425°F/Fan 200°C/Gas Mark 7.

- Drain the pasta shapes and blend into the chicken and tomato sauce. Move to a shallow heatproof dish and sprinkle over the ground mozzarella. Prepare for 15-20 mins until the cheddar is brilliant and gurgling. Serve decorated with basil leaves and a sprinkling of ground dark pepper.

- Halibut with Roasted Tomatoes (Oven-Roasted) and Basil with Tapenade

Ingredients:

250g cherry tomatoes, split; 2 tbsp olive oil; Salt and naturally ground dark pepper; 2 x 200g halibut steaks; 1 clove garlic, stripped and meagerly cut; 1-2 tablespoons olive tapenade (olive glue); Basil leaves.

Directions:

- Set the stove to Gas Mark 3 or 160°C.

- Put the cherry tomatoes in a broiling plate, sprinkle more than 1 tbsp of the oil and season. Heat in the grill for 35 mins.

- Increase the stove temperature to Gas Mark 6 or 200°C.

- Season the halibut steaks and spot in the plate with the cherry tomatoes. Dissipate the garlic over the tomatoes and sprinkle the fish with the rest of the oil.

- Bake the fish for 15-20 mins, until cooked through.

- Serve with the tapenade and basil leaves.

- Prawn Linguine Recipe

Ingredients:

400g linguine; 2tbsp additional virgin olive oil; 2 red chilies, deseeded and finely hacked; 2 lemons, get-up-and-go and squeeze; 3 cloves garlic; 300g crude ruler prawns, stripped; Freshly broke dark pepper; Handful or new coriander leaves, generally slashed.

Guidelines:

147

- Bring an enormous container of water to a bubble. Include the linguine, and cook until still somewhat firm. Channel.

- Heat the oil in an enormous container and include the bean stew, lemon pizzazz, and garlic. Cook for 2 minutes at that point include the prawns. Cook for 2-3mins or until the prawns has turned pink. Include the lemon squeeze and season with pepper.

- Add the linguine to the skillet and hurl altogether. Present with fresh parsley.

- Black pasta with cherry tomatoes and prawns

Ingredients:

250g dark squid ink spaghetti or linguine; 1tbsp olive oil; 300g cherry tomatoes, split; 1 clove garlic, squashed; Juice and pizzazz of 1 lemon; 300g shrimp or prawns; Small pack generally hacked parsley

Directions:

- Cook the pasta as per bundle guidelines, when cooked channel, shower over olive oil, and put in a safe spot.

- While the pasta is cooking heat the oil in a skillet over medium warmth. Cook the tomatoes for 5mins, at that point include the garlic and cook for one more moment. Mix in the prawns and fry until cooked through.

- Add the depleted pasta to the skillet and season well. Mix in the lemon pizzazz and juice to taste. Top with parsley to serve.

- Vegan Pesto Pasta Salad

Ingredients:

Veggie lover Walnut Pesto: 1 cup child arugula; 1 cup new basil; 1/3 cup extra-virgin olive oil; juice of one lemon; 1 clove garlic; 1/4 teaspoon ocean salt (more to taste); 1/2 cup raw pecans.

Pasta Salad: 1-pound rotini pasta (I utilized GF dark colored rice + quinoa pasta); 1 cup solidified peas, defrosted; 1 cup slashed cherry tomatoes; 1 cup crisp infant arugula; 1/4 cup pecans, toasted and cleaved; ocean salt and pepper, to taste; 1 Tablespoon olive oil.

Directions:

- Make pesto sauce by including arugula, basil, oil, lemon juice, garlic and salt in the bowl of a nourishment processor (offshoot connection) and preparing until smooth. Include the pecans and heartbeat until the pecans are ground to desired consistency. Put in a safe spot.

- Cook pasta, as indicated by bundle guidelines. Wash with cold water and channel. Give the pasta a chance to cool for around 5-10 minutes. Add pasta to a massive plate of mixed greens bowl and hurl with defrosted peas, tomatoes, toasted arugula pecans, and olive oil. Include pesto, beginning with ½ cup. Taste and include more pesto on the off chance that you'd like. I like my noodles covered, so I utilized all the pesto. Taste and season generously with salt and pepper. Pasta plate of mixed greens can be served promptly, cold or at room temperature.

- Kale and Red Pepper Shakshuka

Ingredients:

1 tablespoon olive oil; 1 little yellow onion, diced; 1 medium red ringer peppers, cut into slender strips; 2 cloves garlic, minced; 2 cups new picked kale, slashed; 1 tablespoon red wine; 1 teaspoon Italian flavoring; 1/2 teaspoon dark pepper; 1/4 teaspoon simmered red pepper pieces; 1/4 teaspoon salt, to taste; 2 14 ounce jars of diced tomatoes, no-additional salt; 4 huge eggs.

Guidelines:
- Heat olive oil in a large nonstick skillet (like a cast-iron dish) over medium warmth.

- Add onions and cook 2-3 minutes.

- Add the chime pepper and cook an extra 5 minutes, mixing as often as possible until mollified.

- Stir in the minced garlic.

- Add kale by the bunches until it is altogether shriveled.

- Deglaze the container with the red wine, mixing as often as possible for 60 seconds.

- Stir in the Italian flavoring, dark pepper, squashed red pepper, and salt.

- Add the diced tomatoes and blend well until all fixings are consolidated.

- Turn the warmth to medium, spread, and let cook for 5 minutes.

- Remove the top and make four wells in the blend.

- Gently include a split egg into each well.

- Cover again and cook for an extra 6 minutes, or until the white is firm and yolk is set.

- Remove from warmth and appreciate!

- Chickpea and Vegetable Coconut Curry

Ingredients:

1 tablespoon extra-virgin olive oil; 1 red onion, meagerly cut; 1 red chime pepper, daintily cut; 1 tablespoon crisp ginger, minced; 3 garlic cloves, minced; 1 little head cauliflower, cut into reduced down florets; 2 teaspoons chile powder; 1 teaspoon ground coriander; 3 tablespoons red curry glue; One 14-ounce would coconut be able to drain; 1 lime, divided; One 28-ounce can cooked chickpeas; 1½ cups solidified peas; Salt and naturally ground dark pepper; Steamed rice, for serving; ¼ cup hacked new cilantro; 4 scallions, meagerly cut.

Directions:

- In a huge pot, heat the olive oil over medium warmth. Include the onion and ringer pepper, and sauté until about delicate, 4 to 5 minutes. Include the ginger and garlic, and sauté until fragrant, around one moment.

- Add the cauliflower and hurl well to join. Mix in the chili powder, coriander, and red curry glue, and cook until the entire blend obscures somewhat one moment.

- Stir in the coconut milk and carry the blend to a stew over medium-low heat. Spread the pot and keep on stewing until the cauliflower is delicate, 8 to 10 minutes.

- Remove the cover and crush lime juice into the curry, blending admirably to consolidate. Include the chickpeas and peas, season with salt and pepper, and take the blend back to a stew.

- Serve with rice, whenever wanted. Embellishment each bit with one tablespoon cilantro and one tablespoon scallions.

- Baked Sesame-Ginger Salmon in Parchment

Ingredients:

1 teaspoon sesame oil; 2 tablespoons soy sauce; 2 tablespoons ground crisp ginger; 1 teaspoon garlic powder; 2 tablespoons nectar; Pinch of red-pepper pieces; 2 huge zucchini, divided the long way and meagerly cut; 1 red onion, split and daintily cut; 1 lime, quartered; Four 6-ounce skinless salmon filets; 4 teaspoons sesame seeds.

Guidelines:

- Preheat the grill to 350°F. Get ready four bits of material (around 15 by 17 inches). Overlay each piece fifty-fifty to make a wrinkle, at that point unfurl and put in a safe spot.

- In a little bowl, whisk the sesame oil with the soy sauce, ginger, garlic powder, nectar, and red-pepper pieces to consolidate.

- Build the material bundles each in turn. One side of a bit of material, place a fourth of the zucchini in an even layer and top with a fourth of the red onion. Press one of the lime portions liberally over the vegetables.

- Place a salmon filet over the vegetables. Brush the salmon liberally with the soy sauce blend and top with one teaspoon sesame seeds.

- Fold the vacant side of the material over the salmon and afterward overlap the two edges internal toward the salmon, making a few wrinkles to seal the bundle completely.

- Repeat with the rest of the material and fixings. Move the readied bundles to a heating sheet and prepare until the salmon is thoroughly cooked 16 to 18 minutes.

- To serve, expel the fish and veggies from the bundles and move to plates, or cut cuts in the highest point of the material and serve in the paper. Serve right away.

Dessert Recipes in the Mediterranean Diet

- Olive Oil Chocolate Chip Cookie Recipe

Ingredients:

1 cup additional virgin olive oil; 1 tablespoon vanilla concentrate; 3/4 cup granulated sugar

3/4 cup brilliant darker sugar; 1 teaspoon in addition to extra for trimming Kosher salt; 1 huge egg; 2 cups universally handy flour; 1/2 teaspoon preparing pop; 2 cups semisweet chocolate chips.

Guidelines:

- Preheat the grill to 350 degrees F, and line two preparing sheets with material paper. Put in a safe spot.

- Add the olive oil, vanilla, the two sugars and the one teaspoon of salt, to an enormous blending bowl. Blend until you have a smooth consistency.

- Now blend in the egg. Mix until it's smooth once more.

- Add the flour and heating soft drink to the bowl and blend just until it's completely fused and you don't perceive any dry spots of starch.

- Fold in the chocolate chips.

- Use your hand to shape the hitter into balls, around two tablespoons each. (Your side will be oily from the oil; however, I find for this formula, hands are ideal.) Add the molded chunks of the player to the material lined heating sheets as you go. They ought to have at any rate 2-crawls between them, around twelve for each layer.

- Use the palm of your hand to straighten the bundles of hitter, just about midway delicately.

- Then gently sprinkle everyone with Kosher salt.

- Place the heating sheets in the preheated 350-degree F broiler until the treats are brilliant dark-colored along the edges, 10 to 12 minutes. Give them a chance to cool on the preparing sheet for around 5 minutes, at that point place them on a cooling rack to come to room temperature.

- Olive Oil Brownies Made with Greek Yogurt

Ingredients:

1/4 cup olive oil; 1/4 cup low-fat Greek yogurt; 3/4 cup sugar; 1 teaspoon vanilla concentrate; 2 eggs; 1/2 cup flour; 1/3 cup cocoa powder (you can include 1-2 tablespoons progressively); 1/4 teaspoon heating powder; 1/4 teaspoon salt; 1/3 cup slashed pecans.

Directions:
- Preheat the stove at 350 degrees Fahrenheit (180 degrees Celsius)

- In a bowl mix the olive oil and sugar well with a large spoon until smooth. Include vanilla and blend well.

- Beat the eggs in a little bowl and add to the olive oil blend and blend well.

- Add the yogurt and blend well.

- In another bowl mix the flour, cocoa powder, salt, and heating powder. Add to olive oil blend and blend well.

- Incorporate the nuts and blend once more.

- Line a 9-inch square skillet (22 cm) with wax paper and cautiously pour the brownie blend in the dish, smooth the top with a spatula.

- Bake for around 25 minutes.

- Let it cool totally, evacuate the wax paper and cut in squares.

- Greek Yogurt Chocolate Mousse

Ingredients:

180ml/3/4 cup milk; 100g/3 1/2 oz dull chocolate; 500ml/2 cups greek yogurt; 1 tbsp nectar or maple syrup; 1/2 tsp vanilla concentrate.

Guidance:

- Pour the milk into a pan and include the chocolate, either ground or finely slashed or shaved. Delicately heat the milk until the chocolate liquefies, being mindful so as not to allow it to bubble. When the chocolate and milk have completely consolidated, include the nectar and vanilla concentrate and blend well.

- Spoon the greek yogurt into a large bowl and pour the chocolate blend on top. Combine a long time before moving to individual dishes, ramekins, or glasses.

- Chill in the ice chest for 2 hours. Present with a little spoonful of greek yogurt and some new raspberries.

- The chocolate mousse will keep in the ice chest for two days.

- Italian Apple Olive Oil Cake

Ingredients:

2 enormous Gala apples, stripped and hacked as finely as would be prudent; Orange juice to absorb apples; 3 cups universally handy flour; 1/2 tsp ground cinnamon; 1/2 tsp ground nutmeg; 1 tsp preparing powder; 1 tsp heating pop; 1 cup sugar; 1 cup Private Reserve additional virgin olive oil; 2 huge eggs; 2/3 cup gold raisins, absorbed warm water for 15 minutes and afterward depleted well; Confectioner's sugar for cleaning.

Guidelines:

- Preheat grill to 350 degrees F.

- Place the slashed apples in a bowl and include squeezed orange; only enough squeeze to hurl and cover apples to avoid sautéing.

- In a large combining bowl filter the flour, cinnamon, nutmeg, preparing powder and heating pop. Put in a safe spot for the time being.

- In the bowl of a stand blender fitted with a whisk, include sugar and additional virgin olive oil. Blend on low for 2 minutes until well-consolidated

- While the blender is on, include the eggs, each in turn, and keep on blending an additional 2 minutes until blend increments in volume (it ought to be thicker yet runny)

- In the huge bowl with the dry fixings, make a well in the center of the flour blend. Include the wet mixture (the sugar and olive oil mixture) into the well. Utilizing a wooden spoon, mix until mixed; it will be a thick hitter (don't add anything to relax it).

- Drain raisins (which have been absorbing water) totally; and free apples of overabundance juice. Add the two grapes and apples to the player and blend with a spoon until well-joined. Once more, the hitter will be genuinely thick.

- Line a 9-inch cake dish with material paper. Spoon thick player into the bowl, and level the top with the back of your wooden spoon.

157

- Bake in 350 degrees F for 45 minutes or until an embedded tooth choose wooden stick confesses all.

- Cool totally in the dish. Whenever prepared, lift material to exchange cake into a serving dish. Residue with confectioner's sugar. On the other hand, heat some dull nectar to serve on top.

- Blueberry Muffins prepared with Olive Oil.

Ingredients:

Dry fixings: 2 cups generally useful flour; 2 cups entire wheat flour; 2/3 cup sugar; 6 teaspoons heating powder; 1 teaspoon salt; 2 cups blueberries (defrost, whenever solidified)

Wet fixings: 2 eggs; 2/3 cup olive oil; 2 cups milk (of your decision).

Directions:

- Preheat stove to 400 degrees F.

- Combine dry fixings in a bowl. Blend well. Mix in blueberries.

- Combine wet fixings in a little bowl.

- Add wet fixings to dry. Blend just until everything is fused (don't overmix).

- Fill oiled stove tins with biscuit blend.

- Bake for around 18 minutes or until a blade or toothpick tells the truth.

- Honey Almond Ricotta Spread with Peaches

Ingredients:

FOR THE RICOTTA SPREAD: 1 cup whole milk ricotta; 1/2 cup Fisher Sliced Almonds; 1/4 teaspoon almond extricate; 1 teaspoon nectar; pizzazz from an orange, discretionary.

FOR SERVING: hearty entire grain toast, English biscuit or bagel; cut peaches; additional Fisher cut almonds; extra nectar for showering.

Directions:

- Combine ricotta, almonds, and almond remove in a medium measured blending bowl and tenderly mix to consolidate. Move to a serving bowl and sprinkle with extra cut almonds and shower with a teaspoon of nectar.

- To serve, toast your bread. Spread one tablespoon of ricotta spread on each bit of bread. Top with cut peaches, cut almonds and nectar.

- Lemon Olive Oil Cake

Ingredients:

For the cake: 1 cup unsweetened almond milk; 1 tablespoon lemon pizzazz; 1 tablespoon lemon juice; 3/4 cup turbinado sugar; 1/3 cup olive oil; 2 cups entire wheat baked good flour; 1 teaspoon preparing pop; 1/2 teaspoon Salt.

For the coating: 1 cup powdered sugar; 1-2 tablespoons lemon juice; 1/2 teaspoon vanilla concentrate.

Guidelines:

To make the cake:

- Preheat stove to 350 degrees. Line a 9-inch portion dish with material paper and coat with nonstick cooking shower.

- To make veggie-lover buttermilk, in a little bowl whisk together almond milk, lemon pizzazz, and one tablespoon lemon juice. Put aside to mix for 5 minutes

- Meanwhile, whisk together sugar and olive oil in a huge bowl until velvety. Speed in buttermilk blend.

- In a medium bowl, consolidate flour, heating pop, and salt. Crease into buttermilk blend and mix until fused.

- Pour hitter into arranged skillet and smooth the top. Prepare until a toothpick embedded tells the truth with a couple of pieces connected, around 45 minutes.

- Remove from grill and cool in any event 10 minutes in the skillet. Expel to a cooling rack set over a heating sheet and chill totally.

To make the coating:

1. Whisk together staying powdered sugar, lemon juice, and vanilla until smooth. Pour over cooled cake, enabling abundance to dribble off the cake onto the preparing sheet underneath.

- Easy Roasted Fruit Recipe

Ingredients:

Four peaches, stripped and cut; 1/2 cups new blueberries; 1/8 teaspoon ground cinnamon; 3 tablespoons darker sugar.

Directions:

1. Preheat stove to 350-degrees F.

2. Spread cut peaches and blueberries in prepared dish. Sprinkled with cinnamon and darker sugar.

3. Bake at 350-degrees F for around 20 minutes, at that point change broiler settings to a low cook and sear for approximately 5 minutes, or until bubbly.

4. Serve warm, or let cool, spread and refrigerate.

- Fig Almond Olive Oil Cake

Ingredients:

2 Tablespoons/30ml crisp lemon squeeze; The pizzazz of 1 little or a significant portion of a large lemon; ¼ cup/84g nectar; ¼ cup/60ml additional virgin olive oil; 2 enormous eggs; A touch of salt; 1 ½ cups/168g fine almond flour; 1 ½ tsp preparing powder; 8-10 new figs, cut.

Directions:

1. Heat the stove to 350° F. Oil an 8-inch cake container and line the base with material paper.

2. In a huge bowl whisk together the lemon juice, lemon pizzazz, nectar, olive oil, eggs, and salt. Include the almond flour and heating powder; whisk again until joined.

3. Pour the hitter into the readied container and top with fig cuts. Heat for around 35 minutes, until the top is brilliant and focus is set. Move the cake to a rack and let cool.

4. Run a blade around the edge of the dish, modify cake onto a cooling rack, and let cool totally.

• Maple Vanilla Baked Pears

Ingredients:

4 D'Anjou pears (otherwise known as Anjou pears); 1/2 cup (120ml) pure maple syrup; 1/4 teaspoon ground cinnamon; 1 teaspoon unadulterated vanilla concentrate; discretionary fixings: maple walnut granola, Greek yogurt.

Guidelines:

1. Preheat grill to 375°F (190°C). I don't line my preparing sheet when I make these, yet you completely can with material or a silicone heating mat.

2. Cut pears into equal parts, at that point cut a little fragment off the underside, so the pears sit level when set up standing on the preparing sheet. Utilizing a large or medium treat scoop or melon hotshot (or even a teaspoon), center out the seeds. Mastermind pears, looking up, on the heating sheet. Sprinkle equally with cinnamon–don't hesitate to include more cinnamon if you'd like.

3. Whisk the maple syrup and vanilla concentrate together in a little bowl. Sprinkle the vast majority, all things considered, over the pears, holding around 2 Tablespoons for after the pears are done the heating.

4. Bake pears for around 25 minutes until delicate and softly sautéed on the edges. Expel from the stove and promptly shower with outstanding maple syrup blend. Serve warm with granola and yogurt. The store remains in the cooler for as long as five days.

www.ingramcontent.com/pod-product-compliance
Lightning Source LLC
Chambersburg PA
CBHW061346250726
48657CB00004B/1355